Tobacco and Areca Nut

Tobacco and Areca Nut

V M SIVARAMAKRISHNAN

MA PhD DSc

Formerly Head, Isotope Division, Cancer Institute, Chennai

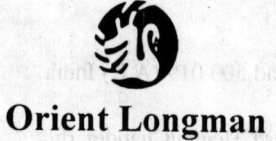

Orient Longman

Orient Longman Limited

Registered Office
3-6-272 Himayatnagar, Hyderabad 500 019 (A.P.) India

Other Offices
Bangalore/Bhopal/Bhubaneshwar/Calcutta/Chandigarh/
Chennai/Ernakulam/Guwahati/Hyderabad/Jaipur/
Lucknow/Mumbai/New Delhi/Patna

© Orient Longman Ltd 2001
First published 2001

ISBN 81 250 2013 6

Typeset by
Nexus Graphics
Chennai 600 020

Printed at
Cubico Press
Chennai 600 014

Published by
Orient Longman Limited
160 Anna Salai
Chennai 600 002

Preface

Tobacco consumption habits in Asia, particularly in India are very different from those in the West. While around 95 per cent of westerners smoke cigarettes, cigarettes account for only 20 per cent of the tobacco consumption in India. Most Indians (80 per cent) smoke bidis. The hookah which is popular in north India and the Middle East, is virtually unknown in the West. Most westerners chew tobacco, with flavouring, or in the powdered form as snuff (a phenomenon known as snuff dipping). A wide variety of chewing practices exist in India and other Asian countries, making use of tobacco, betel leaves, areca nut and slaked lime, in various combinations. The biological effects of all these smoking and chewing habits differ considerably. Numerous books deal with smoking and chewing practices in the West. However, they are not very relevant to India, as they do not deal with tobacco consumption habits (such as smoking bidis or chewing betel quid and areca nut), which are peculiar to India alone. As such, a separate book on smoking and chewing practices in India, is warranted. This book has been written to fulfil that need. It covers all aspects of smoking and chewing habits in India, and those in some of its neighbouring countries.

The book is divided into six sections. The first four chapters, comprising Section I, give a historical account of the discovery of tobacco by Columbus among native Americans in North America, and of the spread of tobacco from North America through Europe into India and other countries. Smoking and chewing practices in various countries are also described. The second section is exclusively devoted to the role of tobacco in the Indian economy, the cultivation of various types of tobacco in different parts of India, the manufacture of tobacco products, the excise duty raised, and the export and foreign exchange earned from tobacco. In Section III the active chemicals present in tobacco, tobacco smoke and areca nut, and their biological effects within the body are discussed.

The biological effects of smoking and chewing tobacco are described in the chapters in Section IV. The chapters deal with harmful effects of smoking on the respiratory and cardiovascular systems, on pregnant women, on women and children and through passive smoking are enumerated. The recently discovered beneficial effects of smoking and the psychological comfort and pleasures enjoyed by smokers (the root cause of persistent smoking) are dealt with in two separate chapters. The harmful effects of chewing, the induction of oral cancer by tobacco, and of the pre-cancers, leucoplakia and oral submucous fibrosis by areca nut preparations, are described separately.

Section V is concerned with tobacco control programmes around the world and their success or failure. It also explores the problems encountered when a smoker tries to quit smoking, the various cessation techniques available to help smokers quit, and how they have been successfully employed in the U.K. and the U.S.A, resulting in progressive decline in smoking and in lung cancer. The difficulties likely to be faced in India in trying to implement any large-scale tobacco control programme are also dealt with. The efforts of the Central Tobacco Research Institute, Rajahmundry, in trying to lower the tar and nicotine yields of cigarettes and bidis, and in finding alternative crops for tobacco; and the large-scale interventional studies carried out for 27 years by the Basic Dental Research Unit and Tata Institute of Fundamental Research, Mumbai, are also described in detail. The last mentioned interventional studies have phenomenal information on smoking and chewing practices in India. In the last chapter we discuss the possible state of affairs in India if the present trends in smoking and chewing tobacco continue unchecked.

In writing this book, I have consulted a number of books and papers have and sought information from various quarters. Further information and constructive criticism on the various topics discussed in this book are welcome, particularly from developing countries in Asia, Africa and South America, so that a revised and enlarged edition of this book, encompassing the whole world, can be brought out, with equal emphasis on developed and developing countries.

V.M. Sivaramakrishnan
M.A. Ph.D. D.Sc.

Contents

Acknowledgements

The author has been helped by a number of people, while writing this book. While it is not possible to acknowledge all of them individually, he would like to thank in particular:

1. Dr. Prakash C. Gupta of the Tata Institute for Fundamental Research, Mumbai, for gifting him the two books, *Control of Tobacco-related Cancers and Other Diseases* and *Tobacco and Health: The Indian Scene*, and a number of reprints on interventional studies;

2. Dr. Fali S. Mehta, Tata Institute of Fundamental Research, Mumbai for his book *Tobacco-related Oral Muscosal Lesions and Conditions in India*;

3. Dr. S. Kori, Director, Directorate of Tobacco Development, Govt. of India, for his publications, *Status paper on Tobacco, 1997*, *Role of Tobacco in Indian Economy*, and others;

4. Dr. S. Ramana, Central Tobacco Research Institute, Rajahmundry, for the booklet, *Tobacco Production Technology*;

5. The American Cancer Society, for its publications *Textbook of Clinical Oncology*, *Cancer: Facts and Figures*, and pamphlets on smoking; and

6. Shri A. Krishnamoorthy, Vice-Chairman, Amalgamations Ltd., for the book *A Comprehensive Text Book of Oncology*, in two volumes, by A.R. Moosa et al.

The financial assistance from the Department of Science and Technology, Govt. of India, is gratefully acknowledged. The author is very thankful to the Madras Science Foundation, particularly to the President, Prof. T.S. Sadasivan, and the Secretary, Prof. T.N. Ananthakrishnan, for sponsoring his application to the D.S.T. for the grant-in-aid, even before he was elected a fellow.

Dedication

Dedicated in fond memory, to my teachers who made me what I am today:

Mr. R. Subbaiyer (Headmaster, Hindu Primary School, Chennai)

Janab Syed Gafoor Shah Sahib Bahadur (Headmaster, Muslim High School, Chennai)

Professor A.C. Joseph (Professor of Chemistry, St. Joseph's College, Tiruchi)

Professor M.V. Sitaraman (Professor of Chemistry, Presidency College, Chennai)

Professor P.S. Sarma (Professor of Biochemistry, University of Madras, Chennai)

Dr. Granville C. Kyker (Chief, Biochemistry Department, ORINS Medical Divison, Oak Ridge, U.S.A.)

Professor Peter Alexander (Professor of Radiobiology, Chester Beatty Research Institute, London, U.K.)

1 The Discovery and Spread of Tobacco

Tobacco (*Nicotiana tabacum*) is a member of the *Solanaceae* family to which the nutritious tomato and potato, the decorative winter cherry and the petunia also belong. The tobacco leaves contain nicotine, a plant alkaloid. Tobacco is a native of North America. Native Americans used tobacco in a number of ways. They often chewed the leaves to relieve hunger and thirst. They also inhaled powdered tobacco ('snuff') to clear the nasal passage, and smoked rolled up tobacco leaves, to relieve fatigue.

The snuff used by native Americans was inhaled though a Y-shaped tube called 'Tobago', or 'Tabaca' in Spanish, hence the name 'tobacco'. They also used tobacco for a variety of medicinal purposes – to relieve toothache, to treat skin wounds, and insect bite, to help digestion by chewing bits of leaves, to treat cold and asthma by inhaling snuff.

When Columbus landed in North America in 1492, he noticed that tobacco could be intoxicating. His followers were quick to see the potential value of tobacco leaves, and brought some to Europe. Raleigh introduced tobacco in England in 1585–86, and did much to popularise smoking for pleasure. The French ambassador to Portugal, Jean Nicot, brought some tobacco leaves to the French court for medicinal purposes. The tobacco plant **Nicotiana tabacum** has been named after him. There was initially some vehement opposition to tobacco in some countries. King James I of England despised smoking, describing it in the most contemptuous terms. Murad the Cruel of Turkey, even went to the extent of hanging people who smoked. The rulers of Russia and Japan also inflicted severe punishments on smokers. Tobacco, however, survived in all the European countries. By the end of the sixteenth century, tobacco cultivation and the use of tobacco leaves for medicinal purposes became widespread all over Europe.

Initially, smoking pipes and cigars was popular in Europe and America. The pipe was brought from America into Europe by sailors. Used by professionals and academicians, they were considered to be 'comforting, homely and inspiring'.

Cigars were considered highly respectable, a sign of affluence, sophistication and aristocracy and 'a feast for the senses'. During the seventeenth century, smoking pipes became very popular throughout Europe.

The nineteenth century saw the birth of the cigarette. Cigarettes are more convenient to use, being inexpensive and ideal for mass production. They are made from fine cut tobacco, wrapped in paper. The cigarette tobacco is a blend of different grades of flue-cured Virginia, Burley, Maryland, and air-cured tobacco. The first cigarette making machine was installed in Havana, Cuba, in 1853. From here, it spread to the American colonies, and then to England (London) and Europe. The availability of cheap cigarettes in abundance led to a phenomenal increase in the number of smokers in these countries. Though the pipe and the cigar are still used in the West, cigarettes seem to be the most popular form of smoking today.

The habit of chewing tobacco also originated in Central and South America. Plain tobacco alone is now only chewed in western countries, and in some developing countries. Chewing tobacco was once very popular in North America and in Europe, in the eighteenth and nineteenth centuries, but became less popular after government regulations against spitting were introduced. Cigarettes, which then became available, were soon adopted as inexpensive substitutes. This led to a decline in tobacco chewing in North America till about 1980.

In the West, tobacco chewing is practised almost exclusively by men of all classes in society. It is mainly available in three forms – firm plug or moist plug tobacco, loose leaf tobacco, and twist (roll) tobacco.

Plug or pressed leaf tobacco is made from enriched tobacco leaves or leaf fragments, wrapped in fine tobacco and pressed into flat bars or rolls. The plug can either be firm or moist, depending on the moisture content. Loose leaf tobacco is made from fermented cigar leaf tobacco to which sugar and flavouring agent are added. It is sold as loose pieces or cut strips. Twist or roll tobacco is made of cured leaf, which has been treated with flavouring agents. The tobacco is held in the buccal or labial sulcus (mandibular groove) for hours and chewed from time to time. Two terms are used to describe the size of the tobacco chewed – the chaw and the quid. The chaw is a wad of tobacco, the size of a golf ball. The quid is usually much smaller and is generally held in the mouth and sucked rather than chewed. The tobacco extract is then spat out.

A more recent practice which is causing considerable concern in the U.S.A. is *snuff dipping*, practised by school children and adolescents. It is also common in the Scandinavian countries, particularly Sweden, but generally among the older age group. Dark or Burley tobacco leaves, are used for preparing chewing tobacco, as well as snuff for dipping. These leaves are aged for one to three years, to prepare chewing tobacco, and even longer to prepare snuff. Snuff, made up of finely cut or powdered flavoured tobacco, is available in three types in the West. Dry snuff is sold as a powder. Moist snuff is made from uniformly cut, small particles of flavoured tobacco packed in moist form in flat containers. Fine cut tobacco is made from air- and fire-cured tobacco. It is similar to moist tobacco, but is more coarse.

Snuff dipping requires placing a pinch of snuff or a porous sachet containing snuff in the gingivo-buccal sulcus for hours. Some people even sleep with snuff inside their mouths. In Denmark, the snuff is usually placed inside the lower labial groove; in Sweden, in the upper labial groove; and in the U.S.A., in the mandibular groove. The snuff used in Denmark, Gothenburg snuff is mild and leads only to leukoplakia (whitening of the surface that stays in contact with the tobacco) in the course of time. But the snuff used in the U.S.A., The Copenhagen snuff" contains strong carcinogens and gives rise to oral cancer. The average snuff user consumes about 10–15 grams of tobacco daily.

It will, thus, be seen that, in the West, tobacco is used for the same purposes for which the American Indians used them – smoking, chewing and inhaling, but in a considerably modified manner. About ninety per cent of tobacco is smoked in the form of filter-tip cigarettes and about 4–6 per cent as cigars or in pipes. About 3–6 per cent is chewed and roughly one per cent is used as snuff. The exact amounts and percentages vary slightly from country to country. Thus, about 95 per cent of tobacco consumed is smoked in the West; only about five per cent constitutes 'smokeless tobacco', unburnt tobacco for chewing and as snuff.

2 Smoking Habits in India

A wide variety of smoking practices exist in India. Around 1600 A.D. Portuguese traders brought tobacco, the pipe, and the cigar, into India. The pipe and the cigar underwent considerable modifications in India. The European style pipe gave rise to its Indian counterparts, the *hookli* and the *chilum*. The water pipe, became the *hookah*. From the cigar came the *cheroot*, the *chuta*, and the *dhumti*. Besides these, a unique tobacco product for smoking, the *bidi*, totally unknown in the West, was invented. India now produces and consumes about 85 per cent of the bidis in the world. Bidi is the most popular form of tobacco used in India. Cigarettes came into India much later, around 1900 A.D. The Indian cigarette industry, however, has grown very fast; so the cigarette is now a strong contender to the bidi. To cater to these diverse forms of smoking, tobacco is being cultivated on a large scale in India. India is now the third largest producer of tobacco in the world, after China and the U.S.A. The various forms of smoking practices in India are described in this chapter.

HOOKAH

The hookah is of historical interest. Portuguese merchants introduced tobacco leaves and European style pipes into Bijapur, the glittering capital of the Adil Shahi kingdom. From here, Asad Beg, the moghul ambassador in Bijapur, took a large quantity of tobacco leaves and pipes to the mughal court. He presented Emperor Akbar with some tobacco leaves and a jewel encrusted European style pipe. Out of courtesy and curiosity, Akbar took a few puffs, but his personal physician was worried that tobacco smoke, a hitherto totally unknown substance, might be dangerous. So, he suggested that the smoke be purified by passing it through water, before being inhaled. Thus, the hookah, or water pipe, came into being. It is a modified pipe, with provision for a water receptacle, through which the smoke will pass before being inhaled. Emperor Akbar and many of the nobles and courtiers enjoyed smoking the hookah. Tobacco, became extremely popular among the nobles and later, among the common people too. The practice of chewing tobacco spread all over north India under the mughal influence. The hookah is still popular in northern and eastern India (Uttar Pradesh, Bihar and West Bengal), particularly in rural areas, both among the affluent as well as the poor. It enjoys social respectability among these people. Sharing a hookah represents social acceptance, brotherhood and equality.

However, the hookah is too cumbersome to be carried. So it is now primarily used by women, who stay at home. It is estimated that 1–2 per cent of men, and 17–26 per cent of women use the hookah in these regions, the highest figure of 26 per cent being found in Darbhanga (Bihar) among women.

The hookah consists of four parts (Fig. 2.1). A small bowl at the top is filled with shredded tobacco, moistened with molasses, and burned in charcoal. The base of the bowl is attached to a long wooden stem. This in turn, leads to a receptacle containing water. On one side of this receptacle, is a long, flexible tube through which the tobacco smoke is inhaled. The smoke is drawn through water, which cools and filters it. A wide variety of hookahs are available – from ornamentally carved brass receptacles and bowls, with embroidered smoking tubes to inexpensive clay bowls, and water receptacles made of coconut shell.

HOOKLI

The hookli is a clay pipe, principally used by about 11 per cent of men in the Bhavnagar district of Gujarat. It resembles the pipes used by Europeans. The stem of the hookli is 7–10 cm long and has a mouth piece. Pipes with wooden stems and detachable clay bowls are also used to minimise the heat at the outer stem. Before filling the hookli with tobacco, a pebble or a stone is put into the bowl to prevent the tobacco from getting into the stem while smoking. About 1.5 g of sun-dried tobacco in flake or in powdered form, is moistened with molasses, and stuffed firmly into the bowl. A pipe once lit is smoked frequently. On an average, about 15 g of tobacco is smoked daily. Hookli smoking generates heat that can be felt at the stem.

CHILUM

The chilum is a straight conical pipe, made of clay. It is 10–14 cm long and does not have a mouth piece. It is held vertically, with the wider end at the top. A pebble or a stone is introduced into it to prevent tobacco from entering into one's mouth. The pipe is then completely filled with tobacco, just as in the hookli; and is lit at the top with glowing charcoal. The narrow end of the pipe, which serves as the mouth piece, is covered with a piece of wet cloth, both to filter the smoke, and to prevent the heat from scorching the mouth. Chilum smoking is an exclusively male habit limited to around two per cent of the population in North India. Like hooklis, chilums are also shared by groups. They are made locally, are cheap, and easily available. They are also used for smoking opium and other narcotics.

The hookah, hookli, and chilum are the three forms of pipe smoking practised in certain regions of India. They are all minor forms of smoking, and account for about five per cent of tobacco consumed.

CIGAR

About nine per cent of the tobacco produced in India is used for cigars, cheroots, and chuttas. It is estimated that about 3000 million pieces of these products are made annually in India. Chuttas and cheroots are made from uncut tobacco. Cigars are made out of air-cured, fermented tobacco, usually in factories, and are more expensive than cheroots or chuttas. A cigar consists of a centre core or filler, a middle portion which holds the filler in shape, and an outer wrapper which gives it colour and texture. Cigars have a closed or tapering head. They are milder, more flavoured, and more expensive than cheroots. Three types of tobacco, a filter, a binder and wrapper tobacco, are used to manufacture cigars. In India, a good filler tobacco is also used for binding. Cigars are used mainly in urban areas by affluent people.

CHEROOT

Cheroots are small cigars made of heavy-bodied tobacco. They have no wrapper and contain a single binder. A cheroot has a thick and a thin end, both of which are open. Cheroots are used primarily in Kerala. About 2.7 per cent of villagers around Ernakulam are cheroot smokers.

CHUTTA

Chuttas are coarsely prepared cheroots, used primarily in the Srikakulam and Vishakhapatnam areas of Andhra Pradesh. They are also used (to a lesser extent), in the coastal areas of Tamil Nadu and Orissa. Chuttas are usually home made; prepared by rolling a tobacco leaf

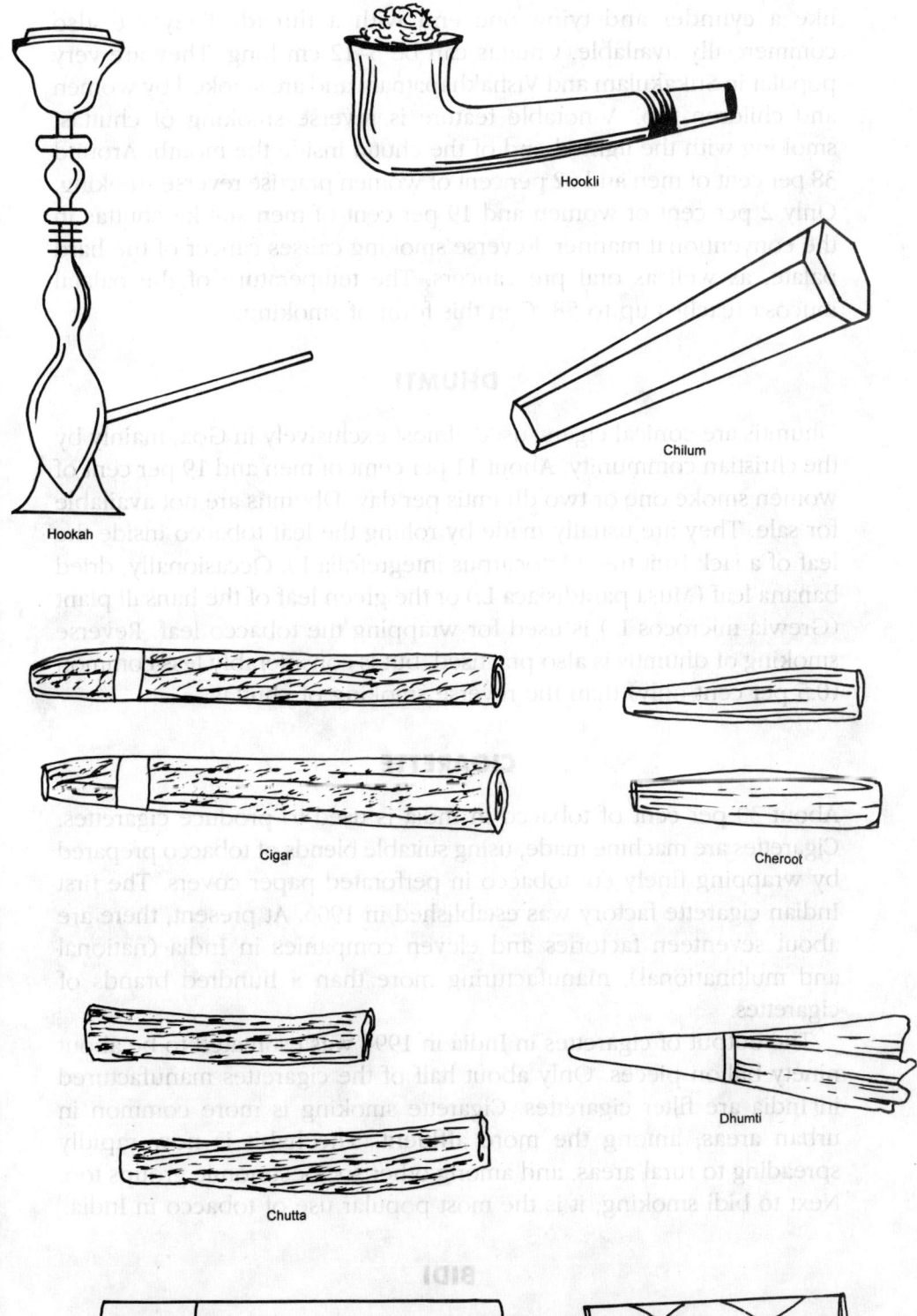

Fig. 2.1 Various forms of smoking practised in India

like a cylinder and tying one end with a thread. They are also commercially available. Chuttas can be 5–12 cm long. They are very popular in Srikakulam and Vishakhapatnam and are smoked by women and children too. A notable feature is reverse smoking of chuttas, smoking with the lighted end of the chutta inside the mouth. Around 38 per cent of men and 62 per cent of women practise reverse smoking. Only 2 per cent of women and 19 per cent of men smoke chuttas in the conventional manner. Reverse smoking causes cancer of the hard palate, as well as oral pre cancers. The temperature of the palatal mucosa reaches up to 58 °C in this form of smoking.

DHUMTI

Dhumtis are conical cigars, used almost exclusively in Goa, mainly by the christian community. About 11 per cemt of men and 19 per cent of women smoke one or two dhumtis per day. Dhumtis are not available for sale. They are usually made by rolling the leaf tobacco inside the leaf of a jack fruit tree (Artocarpus integrefolia L). Occasionally, dried banana leaf (Musa paradisiaca L.) or the green leaf of the hansali plant (Grewia microcos L.) is used for wrapping the tobacco leaf. Reverse smoking of dhumtis is also practised, but is considerably less common (0.5 per cent only) than the reverse smoking of chuttas.

CIGARETTE

About 30 per cent of tobacco in India is used to produce cigarettes. Cigarettes are machine made, using suitable blends of tobacco prepared by wrapping finely cut tobacco in perforated paper covers. The first Indian cigarette factory was established in 1906. At present, there are about seventeen factories and eleven companies in India (national and multinational), manufacturing more than a hundred brands of cigarettes.

The output of cigarettes in India in 1994 was estimated to be about ninety billion pieces. Only about half of the cigarettes manufactured in India are filter cigarettes. Cigarette smoking is more common in urban areas, among the more affluent. The habit is now rapidly spreading to rural areas, and among other socioeconomic groups too. Next to bidi smoking, it is the most popular use of tobacco in India.

BIDI

Bidi smoking is the most popular form of smoking in India. About 34 per cent of the tobacco produced in India is manufactured as bidis.

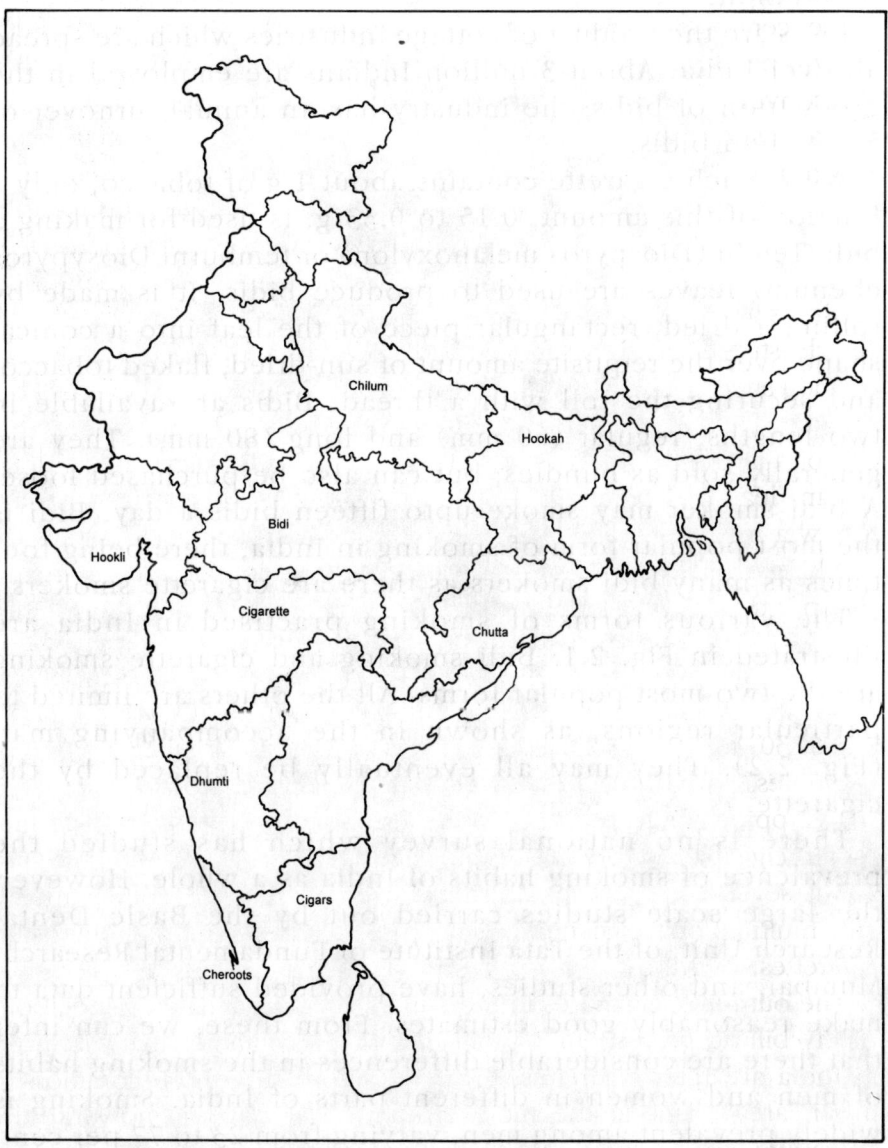

Fig. 2.2   Map showing smoking habits in India (map not to scale)

Bidis probably originated in Bihar, from where they spread to other parts of India and to the neighbouring countries in 1905. India, which produces 550 million bidis every year, now accounts for almost 85 per cent of the world's bidi production.

Bidis are the product of cottage industries which are spread all over India. About 3 million Indians are employed in the production of bidis; the industry has an annual turnover of 550 billion bidis.

While each cigarette contains about 1 g of tobacco, only a fraction of this amount, 0.15 to 0.33 g, is used for making a bidi. Tendu (Diospyros melanoxylon) or temburni Diosypyros ebenum) leaves are used to produce bidis. It is made by rolling a dried, rectangular piece of the leaf into a conical shape over the requisite amount of sun-dried, flaked tobacco, and securing the roll with a thread. Bidis are available in two lengths, regular (60 mm) and long (80 mm). They are generally sold as bundles; but can also be purchased loose. A bidi smoker may smoke upto fifteen bidis a day. Bidi is the most popular form of smoking in India, there being four times as many bidi smokers as there are cigarette smokers.

The various forms of smoking practised in India are illustrated in Fig. 2.1. Bidi smoking and cigarette smoking are the two most popular forms. All the others are limited to particular regions, as shown in the accompanying map (Fig. 2.2). They may all eventually be replaced by the cigarette.

There is no national survey which has studied the prevalence of smoking habits of India as a whole. However, the large scale studies carried out by the Basic Dental Research Unit, of the Tata Institute of Fundamental Research, Mumbai, and other studies, have provided sufficient data to make reasonably good estimates. From these, we can infer that there are considerable differences in the smoking habits of men and women in different parts of India. Smoking is widely prevalent among men, varying from 23 to 77 per cent. In most places, more than 50 per cent of men smoke.

Smoking is relatively uncommon among Indian women except in certain regions. These include ishakhapatnam (in Andhra Pradesh) where about 64 per cent of women smoke chuttas; in Darbhanga (Bihar), where about 28 percent of women smoke hookah, and

13 per cent smoke bidis; in Goa, where about twelve per cent of women smoke bidis and 8 per cent smoke dhumtis. These figures also reveal that compared to the West a much higher percentage of men in India smoke. Smoking is thus a greater menace in India, especially among men.

3 Smokeless Tobacco and Areca Nut

CHEWING HABITS IN INDIA

The term smokeless tobacco, refers to tobacco that is consumed without being burnt. About 18–20 per cent of tobacco in India is chewed, while 80 per cent of it is smoked. In contrast, in the West 95 per cent of tobacco is smoked and only 5 per cent of it is chewed, or used as snuff. The tobacco consumption habits in India have caused a higher incidence of oral cancer, and diseases such as pre cancers, leukoplakia and submucous fibrosis. The following are the typical Indian chewing habits.

BETEL QUID

Betel leaves along with areca nut are often used in hindu religious and social functions. Betrothals and marriage contracts are solemnised by exchanging these. Payments to priests and presentations to others are made reverently, by placing cash over betel leaves and pieces of areca nut.

The practice of chewing betel quid or *paan* is an ancient Indian custom, as old as the practice of smoking tobacco in Central and South America. The essential components of paan are betel leaves, small pieces of areca nut, and slaked lime. One can also add stimulants like catechu (*katha*) and tobacco, and flavouring agents like cinnamon, cardamom, ginger, cloves, menthol, and sugar. In South India a number of shops also sell *beeda*, which is paan decorated with coloured shreds of coconut. Beedas are offered to guests after feasts. Chewing paan stimulates salivation, and aids digestion. Many people, therefore chew beeda after a heavy meal.

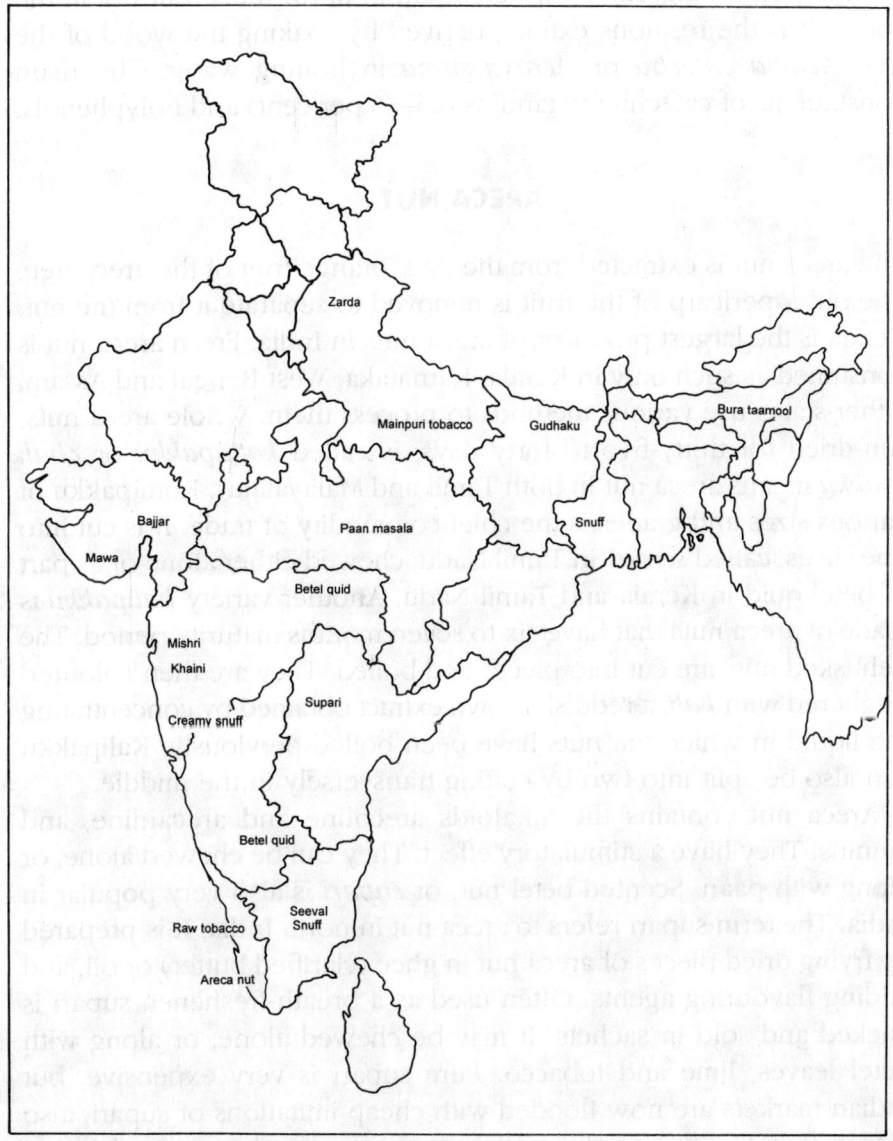

*Fig. 3.1 Map showing smokeless tobacco preparations used in
different regions of India (map not to scale)*

Although chewing paan is a popular habit in India, very few people are addicted to it. A majority of men chew paan only occasionally. Among the various Indian states, paan is most popular in Kerala and Tamil Nadu. Most habitual chewers prefer paan with tobacco. Catechu is an important ingredient of betel quid in north India, but not in the south. It is the resinous extract, derived by soaking the wood of the tree *Acacia catechu* or *Acacia suma* in boiling water. The main constituents of catechu are tannins (25–35 per cent) and polyphenols.

ARECA NUT

The areca nut is extracted from the ripe, orange fruit of the areca tree. The outer pericarp of the fruit is removed to separate it from the nut. Kerala is the largest producer of areca nuts in India. Fresh areca nut is consumed as such only in Kerala, Karnataka, West Bengal and Assam. Other states use various methods to process them. Whole areca nuts, sun-dried for thirty-five to forty days, is called *kottapakku* or *chali* (*pakku* means areca nut in both Tamil and Malayalam). Kottapakku of various sizes and grades is the chief commodity of trade. It is cut into fine slices, called *seeval* in Tamil Nadu, chewed either alone or as part of betel quid in Kerala and Tamil Nadu. Another variety *kalipakku* is made of areca nuts that have six to seven months maturity period. The dehusked nuts are cut into pieces and boiled. They are then coloured bright red with *kali*, a reddish brown extract obtained by concentrating the liquid in which the nuts have been boiled previously. Kalipakku can also be split into two by cutting transversely in the middle.

Areca nut contains the alkaloids arecoline and arecaidine, and tannins. They have a stimulatory effect. They can be chewed alone, or along with paan. Scented betel nut, or *supari* is also very popular in India. The term supari refers to areca nut in north India. It is prepared by frying dried pieces of areca nut in ghee (clarified butter) or oil, and adding flavouring agents. Often used as a breath-freshener, supari is packed and sold in sachets. It may be chewed alone, or along with betel leaves, lime and tobacco. Pure supari is very expensive, but Indian markets are now flooded with cheap imitations of supari, also sold in sachets. The ingredients of these cheaper products are unknown, and could contain items that are injurious to health.

The most widely used areca nut preparation in India is probably *paan masala*, which contains most of the ingredients of paan – areca nut, slaked lime, catechu and spices. It however, does not contain betel leaves, and is hence unperishable. Many brands of paan masala contain tobacco. Sold in attractive packets and tins, they are extremely popular in urban areas and are now becoming popular in rural areas too. Over 150 units exist in north India alone, manufacturing this product, with sales turnover running into crores of rupees. It is also exported to a number of countries.

A fermented form of areca nut, called *taamool* is widely used in Assam. It is prepared by fermenting fresh, ripe, areca nuts and leaves inside a pit lined with straw, for four months. The fermented nut may be slightly infected with fungus. Taamool contains very high levels of arecoline, the areca nut alkaloid which could be the reason for high levels of pharyngeal and esophageal cancers.

An areca nut preparation that is becoming increasingly popular among the youth in Gujarat and its neighbouring areas, is *mawa*. It is a mixture of areca nut shavings (5–6 g) and tobacco (about 0.3 g), sprinkled with a few drops of watery slaked lime. The mixture is rubbed vigorously to make it homogeneous, and any coarse piece of tobacco is removed. Mawa is chewed until it becomes soft, is then transferred into the mandibular groove, and sucked for ten to twenty minutes, until it becomes bland. A variant of mawa, also used in Gujarat is *meetha mawa*. It consists of thin shavings of areca nut, grated coconut, dried fruits and other sweeteners.

TOBACCO

Only about 2–3 per cent of Indians chew plain tobacco – either raw, or finely cut. Most people prefer to use processed tobacco, with betel quid, or slaked lime, or areca nut and slaked lime and flavouring spices. In Kerala, people chew strands of raw tobacco with paan. In Karnataka, women chew tobacco leaves either alone or in paan. Powdered tobacco is chewed either alone, or mixed with jaggery and water. Fried and powdered tobacco along with coriander seeds and other spices, and scented with a resinous oil is used in Orissa, West Bengal and Gujarat. *Pattiwalla, zarda* and *kiwam* are popular tobacco preparations used in northern India. Pattiwalla is sun-cured tobacco, used with or without lime. Zarda which is sold in sachets is prepared by boiling pieces of tobacco leaves with lime and spices until the water evaporates. Colouring and flavouring agents are then mixed to the dry residue. Zarda, which is used in India and in the Arab countries, can be chewed alone, with areca nut, or with paan. Kiwam is prepared by boiling tobacco leaves from which the midribs and veins have been removed in water. Powdered saffron, cardamom, aniseed and musk are then added. The solution is thoroughly mixed and boiled till a thick paste is obtained, from which pellets or granules can be prepared.

Mainpuri tobacco, popular in Mainpuri, Uttar Pradesh, is tobacco mixed with slaked lime, finely cut areca nut, camphor and cloves. About 7 per cent of the villagers in Mainpuri and its surrounding areas use it regularly. Prolonged use of Mainpuri tobacco causes leukoplakia and oral cancer.

Khaini a mixture of sun-dried, powdered tobacco, and slaked lime, is widely used in Maharashtra, Gujarat, Bihar, and Uttar Pradesh. The mixture is prepared by rubbing together powdered tobacco and moistened slaked lime (*chunam*), and is then placed inside the mouth. In Maharashtra and Gujarat, khaini is placed in the premolar region of the mandibular groove, in the lower labial groove in Bihar and Uttar Pradesh, and on the dorsum of the tongue in Singbhum District (Bihar). Khaini is not chewed, but sucked periodically, until it becomes bland. About 0.2 g of the tobacco-lime mixture is consumed at a time several times in a day. It is usually men who use khani, although a small percentage of women also use it in these states.

Thus, a wide variety of tobacco preparations, each one limited to a particular regions, is chewed in India.

TOBACCO PREPARATIONS AS DENTIFRICES

Native Americans used tobacco powder for cleaning their teeth. They also used tobacco to relieve toothache. In some parts of India too, tobacco preparations are used as dentifrices for cleaning teeth. Four such preparations are:
1.   *Mishri* used by women in Maharashtra and Goa,
2.   *Bajjar* commonly used by women in Gujarat,
3.   *Gudhaku* used mainly by women in Bihar, and
4.   *Creamy snuff* used in Goa, primarily by school children.

The use of these preparations are confined to particular localities and can become addictive.

Mishri is prepared by roasting tobacco on a hot metal plate, until it becomes uniformly charred and then powdering it. It is carried in a small metal container by women, who apply it to their teeth and gums. Mishri was initially used only to clean teeth. However, it has now become an addiction, causing people to apply it to their teeth and gums several times a day. It is almost exclusively a female habit; about 39 per cent of women in rural Maharashtra use it.

Bajjar is dry snuff, used by about 14 per cent of women in Gujarat. It is carried in a small, metal container and applied to the teeth and gums with a twig. Gudhaku which is available commercially, is a paste made of tobacco and molasses, and is applied to the teeth and gums with a finger. It is used predominantly by women in Bihar, and other parts of eastern India. Red tooth powder (*lal dant manjan*) is a commercially available dentifrice containing significant amounts of tobacco (about 6 per cent).

Creamy snuff is a commercial preparation, containing mainly tobacco, and resembling toothpaste in consistency. It is marketed in tubes that are similar to toothpaste, and is sold under various brand names. Creamy snuff is advertised as a product possessing antibacterial properties, that protect and strengthen gums and teeth. Though costlier than toothpaste, it has become very popular among school children in Goa, who soon become addicted to it. Some of these children may even use mishri (also called *masheri*). Tobacco chewing habits are more prevalent among boys.

SNUFF

Snuff is finely powdered tobacco that can be used orally or nasally. Scented snuff is often inhaled. Snuff originated in North America, became popular in Europe, and then in other parts of the world, including India.

Only about one per cent of the tobacco consumed in India is used as snuff. It is manufactured mainly in Tamil Nadu, Gujarat and Uttar Pradesh. Chennai (in Tamil Nadu), is an important centre for manufacturing snuff. Thick, pungent tobacco leaves, are usually selected to manufacture snuff.

Bajjar, a kind of dry snuff, is used orally as a dentifrice for cleaning teeth and gums by women in Gujarat. Inhaling snuff, both to clear nasal passages, and as a stimulant, is common mainly in Tamil Nadu and West Bengal. Snuff-dipping, as practised in the West, is practically non-existent in India. Whichever way it is used, snuff is also addictive like all other tobacco products.

The various regions of India, and the different smokeless tobacco preparations used in those regions are depicted in Fig. 3.1.

4 Tobacco Smoking and Chewing Habits in Asia

Tobacco is smoked and chewed in other Asian countries too.These habits resemble those in India more closely than those in the West. Smoking bidis and hookahs, and chewing paan are habits unique to Asia; smoking and chewing practices in Asian countries are more diverse than those among countries in the West. This chapter briefly examines the smoking and chewing habits in Asia.

SMOKING

In the West, women took to cigarettes a few decades ago. In most western countries, the number of men and women who smoke is roughly equal. But this is not so in Asia and Africa. In most Asian countries, smoking is primarily a male habit. In Sri Lanka for example, 54.8 per cent of men smoke, compared to only 0.84 per cent of women. Similarly, in China, while the percentage of men who smoke ranges between 56 per cent and 93 per cent, only about one per cent of women are addicted to smoking. In most other Asian countries, while more than half of the men smoke, the percentage of women doing so is less than ten per cent. There are three notable exceptions to this: in Papua New Guinea and Nepal, about 80 per cent of men and 75 per cent of women smoke as against Malaysia, where only about 18 per cent of men and 2 per cent of women smoke. The percentage of men and women smoking in some countries are presented in Table 4.1.

CIGARETTE

Cigarette smoking is quite popular in third world countries. Their popularity is increasing rapidly, thanks to aggressive promotions by cigarette companies. In Sri Lanka, the cigarette is the most popular form of smoking. About 38 per cent of smokers smoke only cigarettes, while another 32 per cent smoke both cigarettes and bidis. Only about 15 per cent are exclusively bidi smokers. This is in sharp contrast to India, where bidi smokers outnumber cigarette smokers by four to five times. In China, many people smoke the cigarette till only a very small butt is left. This is harmful because it produces leukoplakia in the labial mucosa, similar to leukoplakia caused by smoking hooklis, as seen in the Bhavnagar district of Gujarat.

Table 4.1: Percentage of male and female smokers in some countries

Country	Men (%)	Women (%)
Australia (national)	37	30
Bangladesh (regional)	70	20
Brazil (regional)	54	20
China (regional)	56	1
Egypt	93	1
India		
regional	66	26
urban	29	3
rural	61	7
Indonesia (various regions)	63–75	5–10
Israel (national)	44	30
Malaysia	18	2
Nepal	85	75
Sri Lanka	55	0.8
Pakistan (regional)	44–49	4.6
Papua New Guinea	77–85	76–80
Singapore (national)	51	8.3
Thailand (national)		
Urban	51	4
Rural	70	40
United States (national)	38	30
Zambia (regional)	63	56

Source: World Health Organization. Data selected from WHO report (1986). The percentages may have changed slightly since then.

Bidi

Bidi smoking is common to India, Pakistan, Bangladesh, Nepal, Burma, andSriLanka but is not very well known in the other Asian countries.

Cigar

Cigars are used in various forms in Asian countries, although they are now being replaced by cigarettes. Smoking large cigars is believed to be an American habit. Cheroots, small cigars made of heavy-bodied tobacco with both ends cut off are common in Burma, and are used even by boys. A variant of cheroot, called *keeyo*, is also popular in Thailand. The bark of the keeyo tree (Streblus asper L.) is used to wrap the tobacco mixture, while preparing the keeyo. The characteristic flavour of the keeyo smoke comes from this outer covering. Occasionally, a banana leaf is used to wrap the tobacco. A survey conducted in 1986 in the Chiang Mai area in northern Thailand revealed that a fifth of the people smoked keeyos, and 4.5 per cent smoked 8–10 cm long cigars, made by wrapping very finely cut tobacco inside a corn leaf.

Kreteks, is the most popular cheroot smoked in Indonesia and has been used since 1824. It is made of tobacco, cloves, and cocoa. The smoke from a kretek has a characteristic smell and taste of honey. Kreteks are very cheap, and can be purchased as singles. They last for a long time and extinguish themselves automatically, when placed down. Hence, they are very popular in Indonesia, particularly in rural areas. While being smoked, they often emit a characteristic sound, and send occasional sparks. They yield two to five times as much tar and nicotine as a western cigarette.

Pipe

Pipe smoking is also common in many parts of Asia. Various types of pipes are used. Small European style pipes are used by tribal women in Chiang Mai area in northern Thailand. Elderly persons in China use pipes with very long stems, which helps cool the smoke by the time it reaches the mouth, so that oral lesions are insignificant. Nepalese use clay pipes called *sulpa*, similar to the chilum in Gujarat. Modern and sophisticated European style pipes, made of wood and clay, are also seen in these countries.

Water Pipe

Water pipes, using the principle of the hookah, are used widely in the Middle East, in various other countries in Asia, and in parts of Africa.

It is considered the healthiest form of smoking, since the smoke is filtered of tar and nicotine through water. It is the equivalent of the mildest of cigarettes. Unfortunately, sharing the hookah is reported to help spread tuberculosis.

Water pipes used in different countries are of various designs and sizes, and are known by different names – hookah, goza, hubble-bubble, narghit, and sheesha. They range from small, elegant ones used in Papua New Guinea to large, bulky bamboo water pipes, about one metre long, widely used by the Karen tribes of Thailand.

CHEWING

TOBACCO

Tobacco chewing is quite common in all Asian countries, but only a small percentage of people, 2 to 3 per cent chew plain tobacco. In most of these countries, tobacco is chewed either as a special preparation, or along with betel quid. Almost all these preparations contain slaked lime as an integral component. This makes the preparation slightly alkaline, and allows nicotine to be extracted from the tobacco, and absorbed into the body.

The popular tobacco preparations in India, khaini, zarda and Mainpuri tobacco, have already been described. *Shammah, nass* and *naswar* are similar tobacco preparations used in some South-West Asian countries. Shammah is a mixture of powdered tobacco leaf, carbonate of lime ($CaCO_3$), and unspecified ingredients, and is used in Saudi Arabia. Nass is a mixture of tobacco, ash, cotton or sesame oil, lime and sometimes gum. It is chewed in Iran and Central Asian republics. Naswar is used in Pakistan, Afghanistan, Iran and in the Central Asian republics. It is prepared from sun-dried, powdered tobacco, lime, and indigo, which gives it an attractive colour. In Afghanistan, a small quantity of this finely powdered, homogeneous mixture is placed on the floor of the mouth, and sucked from time to time until bland. Malignant transformation of the floor of the mouth occurs in due course. Naswar is used similarly, in Iran and in the Central Asian republics. In Pakistan, a variant of naswar, is made of a mixture of sun-cured tobacco, ash, slaked lime, water, and flavouring agents such as cardamom oil.

We can thus see that these tobacco preparations are essentially prevalent in India, and in the countries to its west.

BETEL QUID

According to World Health Organization (WHO) report in 1985, countries where significant betel quid chewing is prevalent include India, Pakistan, Nepal, Sri Lanka, Bangladesh, Burma, Malaysia, Singapore, Indonesia, Thailand, Kampuchia, Laos,Vietnam, Philippines, Taiwan, some parts of China, and in Papua New Guines and its associated island groups, such as New Ireland and New Britain.

Betel quid chewing is thus common to the Indian subcontinent and to all countries to its east. The habit probably originated in India and spread eastwards to South-East Asia and Melanesia. Betel quid is also popular among Indians in various parts of the world; the Fiji islands in the Pacific, Tanzania, Kenya and South Africa, the U.K. and the U.S.A. It is estimated that about 300 million to 600 million people habitually chew betel quid.

While in India, most people who chew betel quid also chew tobacco, this is so in only among half the betel quid chewers in Sri Lanka. In Papua New Guinea and other South Pacific Islands, betel quid is chewed without tobacco. In Malaysia *gambir*, prepared from the twig and leaves of the shrub Uncaria gambir, is used as a stimulant in betel quid, instead of the catechu used in India. Processed areca nut is extensively used in India, while in Melanesia, mainly raw areca nut is used.

There are also different ways of chewing the components of betel quid. In India, the mixture is folded with a betel leaf, which is then chewed. In Indonesia, the areca nut pieces and betel leaves are smeared with lime and chewed first, after which tobacco is taken in. In Papua New Guinea, areca nut pieces are chewed first, after which a small amount of lime is placed on the buccal mucosa. Betel leaves are then taken in, and the whole mixture is chewed.

TOBACCO SMOKING AND CHEWING
PRACTICES IN OTHER COUNTRIES

Cheroots are very common in Denmark, particularly among women. When smoked, they can cause leukoplakia in the floor of the mouth. Reverse smoking of cigars or cigarettes, similar to chutta smoking in Srikakulam area, is quite common in many South American countries such as Columbia, Venezuela, the Caribbean, and the Dutch Antilles, and is practised mainly by women. In Sardinia reverse smoking is popular among men. Habitual reverse smoking leads to lesions in the hard palate (roof of the mouth), and can cause cancer.

Smoking tobacco is not popular in Africa. The Bantus in South Africa both chew and dip snuff. The snuff used by them is made from tobacco leaves and wet ash from aloe, or other plant leaves. Oil, lemon juice, and herbs, are sometimes added. This preparation, which is somewhat alkaline, is used by both men and women, who keep it in their lower labial groove. This snuff is mild causing only a yellowish white lesion in that area, but is not carcinogenic.

The Sudanese use a coarse preparation of strong snuff. Like khaini, it is made from finely cut tobacco mixed with slaked lime and kept in the lower labial groove. This results in a malignant transformation in that area.

OTHER FORMS OF SMOKING AND CHEWING

Australian aborigines use *pituri* leaves from the desert shrub *Duboisia hopwoodii*. Chewing pituri also acts as a stimulant, and reduces hunger, fatigue and thirst. Smoking these leaves causes people to become tranquil. Just like tobacco, these leaves contain significant amounts of the alkaloids, nicotine, and nornicotine.

Cocoa leaves are chewed as a powerful stimulant and hunger depressant, mainly in South America, and to a limited extent in India, Sri Lanka and Java. They contain significant quantities of the alkaloid cocaine, a local anesthetic.

Chewing the cola nut is common in Central and West Africa. It is found in the *Cola acuminate*, *Cola verticillara* and *Cola nitida* trees, and contains the alkaloids caffeine and theobromine. It is also a stimulant, relieving fatigue and depressing hunger and thirst.

The leaves of khai shrub (*Cattia edulis*), found in Arabia and East Africa, are chewed by both men and women in all strata of society. It contains pharmacologically active substances including alkaloids, tannins and norpseudoephedrine. All these plants are rich in alkaloids,which are responsible for their biological effects.

Inhaling the smoke from medicinal plants like *Lobella excelsa* and Datura for therapeutic purposes is a very old practice in India. Datura is used to relieve asthma. The twigs of the neem tree (Azadirachta indica) are also used as toothbrush in rural India.

The well known narcotics, opium, derived from poppy (*Papavaer somniferrum*) and marijuana, (*Cannabis sativa*), are used in various ways for psychological and medical treatment. Smoking them produces an exhilarating, tranquillising and occassionally hallucinating effect. Pethidine, and more importantly, oral morphine, derived from opium, are used extensively as painkillers, particularly in diseases like cancer.

5 Tobacco in the Indian Economy

Production of tobacco and tobacco products

Tobacco is an important commercial crop in many countries, including India. It is grown in more than sixty countries in the world. India is the third largest producer of tobacco after China and the U.S.A. The world production of tobacco in 1995 was 6,508 million kg, of which India contributed 587 million kg accounting for 9 per cent of world production. Brazil, Turkey, Zimbabwe, and Malawi are other important tobacco producing countries.

There are about sixty-five known varieties of tobacco, but only two of these, *Nicotiana tabaccum* and *Nicotiana rustica*, are extensively cultivated. Both the varieties are grown in India. Nicotiana tabaccum is grown all over the country, but *Nicotiana rustica* which requires, cooler climate is cultivated primarily in the north and north-eastern states. Andhra Pradesh and Gujarat, are the two largest tobacco producing states, together accounting for three-fourths of tobacco produced. Andhra Pradesh is the principal producer of cigarette tobacco, and Gujarat, of bidi tobacco. Karnataka the third largest tobacco producing state, grows large amounts for both cigarettes and bidis. The production, properties and utilisation of various types of tobacco are described below.

CIGARETTE

Flue-cured Virginia (FCV) tobacco

The main component of cigarettes, is flue-cured Virginia tobacco and is grown in Guntur in Andhra Pradesh and Karnataka. The British settlers first began cultivating Nicotine tabacum in Virginia, after bringing it from the West Indies. Over the years, they managed to cultivate a milder, smoother version of this crop in Europe. By the 1800s, this tobacco began to be flue-cured and processed thus becoming aromatic and colourful. Flue-cured Virginia tobacco, is now an essential ingredient of cigarettes all over the world. Keeping in mind its commercial value, the Pusa Farm in Bihar made a number of unsuccessful attempts to grow this crop. Finally in 1928, the Indian Leaf Tobacco Development (ILTD) company successfully cultivated it, in the black soil area in Guntur, Andhra Pradesh. Flue-cured Virginia (FCV) tobacco then began to be cultivated in other coastal districts of Andhra Pradesh In 1937, the Mysore Tobacco Company began producing flue-cured Virginia tobacco in Karnataka. The area under FCV production in Andhra Pradesh steadily increased to 1,15,000 hectares in 1991–92. Tobacco produced in the black soil region is lemon yellow, comparatively slick, and burns quite well. It is considered a neutral tobacco, and is primarily used for blending. Andhra Pradesh and Karnataka are the two important states producing FCV tobacco in India, Andhra Pradesh accounting for about 80 per cent.

While FCV tobacco raised from black soil can burn well, it is relatively bland, and emits pungent smoke. In 1966-67 therefore, a government sponsored project attempted to grow it in light soils, to get a milder flavour. Certain light soil areas, primarily in Andhra Pradesh and Karnataka, were found suitable, yielding tobacco with a low tar and low nicotine. In terms of filling value, the Karnataka tobacco is on par with the American tobacco.

In 1996, India produced only 108 million kg of FCV tobacco, just about three per cent of world production (4,534 million kg). The largest producer of FCV tobacco is China, accounting for 1,435 million kg in 1996. India stands fifth, after China, U.S.A, Brazil and Zimbabwe.

About forty per cent of the FCV tobacco produced in India is used for producing cigarettes within the country, and the rest is exported. There are about seventeen factories and eleven companies in India which manufacture cigarettes. The cigarette industry is capital-intensive in the organised sector, employing about twenty thousand people in production alone. Lakhs of people are involved in its trade and distribution. India produced 90 billion cigarettes in 1994, about 1.6 per cent of the world output of 5,343 billion. More than a hundred brands of cigarettes are produced in India.

Natu tobacco

Natu or country tobacco (N. tabaccum) is an aromatic type of sun-cured tobacco, produced only in Andhra Pradesh, where it is grown in both black and light soils. It is used for making cheaper brands of cigarettes, and country cheroots. Natu tobacco is also used in pipes, as snuff, or chewed plain.

Burley Tobacco

Burley tobacco is a light air-cured tobacco, used to make cigarettes and pipe mixtures. It is ideal for cigarettes because it has a high nicotine content, and it is five times more efficient in absorbing flavouring agents and other additives.

Only small amounts of Burley tobacco are grown in India. In 1995–96, Andhra Pradesh produced about 3 million to 7 million tonnes of this crop. It is used both for domestic consumption and export. Some brands of cigarettes, such as Charms manufactured in Hyderabad, use Burley tobacco. Indians have only now begun to appreciate the potential of Burley tobacco variety of tobacco or brand. A Brazilian variety, HDBRG, with an annual production of 11 million kg, has now been introduced in Andhra Pradesh.

BIDI TOBACCO

Bidi tobacco is the most important non-Virginia tobacco produced in India. About 190 million to 220 million kg of bidi tobacco are produced annually in India. Gujarat, Karnataka and Maharashtra are the major producers of bidi tobacco, with Gujarat accounting for about 80 per cent, followed by Karnataka (12 per cent), and Maharashtra (8 per cent). Gujarat has the highest productivity of bidi tobacco, with about 1,800 kg per hectare. Tobacco produced in Kaira, on the banks of the Mahi and Sabarmati rivers, is considered very good and used all over the country. In Karnataka, bidi tobacco is produced mainly in the Nipani area of Belgaum district, on the banks of river Krishna. It is considered to be of superior quality, although it has a low yield, only 1,000 kg per hectare.

Bidi smoking is popular primarily in India, Nepal, Bangladesh, Pakistan, Sri Lanka, Burma, Malaysia, and Singapore. India is the largest producer of bidis in the world, producing about 550 billion bidis per year.

The cottage industries of India are the primary producers of bidi, and employ over three million people. The important centres of bidi manufacture are Mangalore, Mysore, Nipani in Karnataka, Nasik, Pune,Tirunelveli in Tamil Nadu,Chennai, Cannanore in Kerala, and Nizamabad, Karimnagar, and Warangal in Andhra Pradesh. Bidis are also produced in Gujarat, Orissa, Uttar Pradesh and West Bengal.

About 300,000 tonnes of tendu leaves are used annually while manufacturing bidis. Being flexible, easily available, and resistant to early decay, these leaves are ideal for wrapping the tobacco. Tendu trees are found in the forests of Madhya Pradesh, Maharashtra, Orissa,

Andhra Pradesh, Bihar and Uttar Pradesh. Madhya Pradesh produces about 50 per cent while Orissa, Maharashtra and Andhra Pradesh together account for about 30 per cent of the leaves used. The tribals collect the leaves, dry them, sort them, and hand them over to state government agencies.

CIGAR AND CHEROOT TOBACCO

There are three types of tobacco used to make cigars – fillers, binders and wrappers. In India, a good filler tobacco is also used as a binder. The filler tobacco for cigars is produced mainly in Dindigul and Tiruchi districts of Tamil Nadu, while good quality wrapper tobacco is grown only in the Cooch Behar district of West Bengal. Cheroots are manufactured mainly from cheroot tobacco, produced in Salem and Coimbatore, in Tamil Nadu. Lanka and natu tobacco grown in Andhra Pradesh are also used to make cheroots.

Cigars and cheroots are traditionally handmade, though cigars can now be manufactured through machines. Because of the increasingly popular cigarette, the cigar industry in India is now confined to Woriyur, Tamil Nadu. The main production centres for cheroots are Madurai and Salem in Tamil Nadu, a number of places in Andhra Pradesh, Sambalpur in Orissa, and Cooch Behar in West Bengal.

HOOKAH TOBACCO

Hookah tobacco is acquired from the *N. rustica* plant, which is produced mainly in northern India. Some *N. tabaccum* varieties are also used for making hookah tobacco. The largest producer of hookah tobacco is Uttar Pradesh (73.3 million kg) followed by Gujarat, Bihar, and West Bengal. The major districts cultivating hookah tobacco are Farrukhabad and Etah in Uttar Pradesh, Kaira and Ahmedabad in Gujarat, Purnia in Bihar, and Cooch Behar, and New Jalpaiguri in West Bengal. Three-fourths of the tobacco grown in West Bengal comes from *N. rustica* plants, the better grades of which are used for chewing. Hookah tobacco is manufactured in a number of places in Uttar Pradesh, in Ahmedabad, Delhi, Chandigarh, and Calcutta.

CHEWING TOBACCO

Chewing tobacco is cultivated in almost all the Indian states. India produces 67.72 million kg of chewing tobacco annually. It is grown in Tamil Nadu, Uttar Pradesh, Gujarat, Bihar, Orissa, and West Bengal. Tamil Nadu, Gujarat and Bihar grow certain varieties of tobacco exclusively for chewing. Other states use this tobacco both for chewing and in the hookah. Coimbatore and Periyar in Tamil Nadu, Farrukhabad in Uttar Pradesh, Vaishali and Samastipur in Bihar, Cooch Behar in West Bengal and Koreput in Orissa are the important chewing tobacco growing districts. A total of 35 million kg of tobacco is chewed annually in India. Three varieties, zarda or flake tobacco, dana or minced tobacco variety and kiwam or tobacco paste are used.

SNUFF

There is no special variety of tobacco grown exclusively for snuff in India. Generally, medium to thick textured leaves with a pungent aroma, are chewed and used as snuff. Tobacco used in hookahs and bidis are also used for making snuff.

Andhra Pradesh, Kerala, Uttar Pradesh, West Bengal, Gujarat, and Punjab are the significant producers of tobacco for snuff. About 11 million to 13 million kg of tobacco is used for making snuff in India.

Snuff is made mostly in Tamil Nadu, Gujarat, Punjab and Uttar Pradesh. In Kerala, Puchakkad tobacco is both chewed and used as snuff. In Gujarat, the important snuff manufacturing centre is Saurashtra. In West Bengal, the Motihari and Vilayati varieties of *N. rustica* tobacco are used as snuff. West Bengal and Tamil Nadu are the primary consumers of snuff. The important snuff manufacturing centres in India are Chennai and Tiruchi in Tamil Nadu; Bhavnagar, Veerangam and Anand in Gujarat; Haridwar in Uttar Pradesh; Pali in Rajasthan; Mangalore in Karnataka; Pune in Maharashtra; and Giddarbha in Punjab.

The regions where different types of tobacco are grown and places where different tobacco products are manufactured are shown in Fig. 5.1.

EXPORT OF TOBACCO AND TOBACCO PRODUCTS

India is one of the leading exporters of tobacco in the world, exporting both raw tobacco, as well as tobacco products. Raw tobacco accounts for 85 per cent of the exports, valued in 1995–96 at Rs. 361.36 crores. India accounts for about 7 per cent of the world export of FCV tobacco. The main importers of Indian tobacco are the U.K. and Russia. Tobacco is also exported to France, Belgium, Netherlands, Germany, Italy and Poland, in Europe; Saudi Arabia, Yemen and United Arab

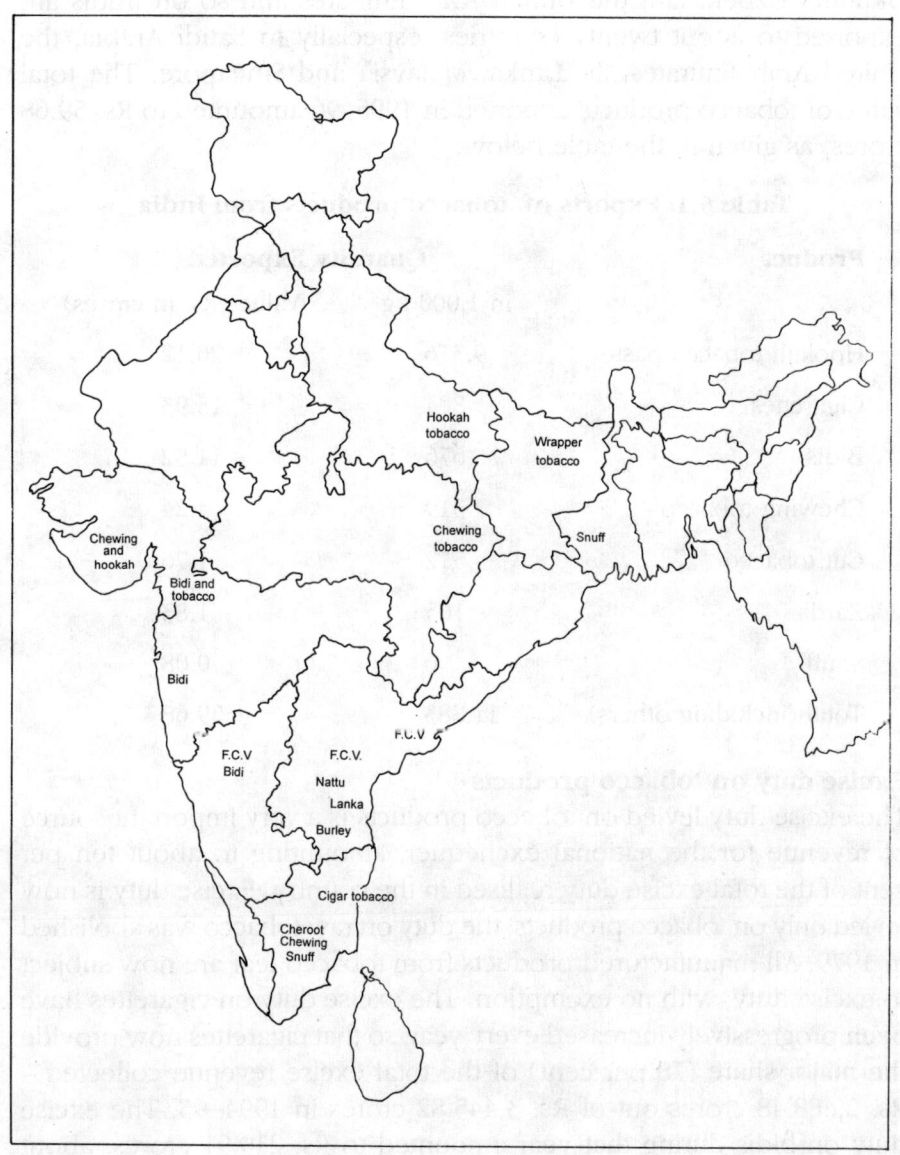

Fig. 5.1   Tobacco map of India (map not to scale)

Emirates in the Middle East; Egypt, Algeria and Libya in Africa; and to
Nepal, Bangladesh and Singapore.

Hookah paste is the major tobacco product exported to the Middle
East, especially to Saudi Arabia. Cigarettes are exported to Russia,
Ukraine, Uzbekistan, the United Arab Emirates and so on. Bidis are
exported to about twenty countries, especially to Saudi Arabia, the
United Arab Emirates, Sri Lanka, Malaysia and Singapore. The total
value of tobacco products exported in 1995–96 amounted to Rs. 59.68
crores, as given in the table below:

Table 5.1: Exports of tobacco products from India

Product	Quantity Exported	
	in 1,000 kg	Value (Rs. in crores)
Hookah tobacco paste	9,376	26.12
Cigarettes	884	13.93
Bidis	676	11.52
Chewing tobacco	319	4.24
Cut tobacco	512	1.76
Zarda	105	1.83
Snuff	6	0.08
Total (including others)	11,883	59.68

Excise duty on tobacco products

The excise duty levied on tobacco products is a very important source
of revenue for the national exchequer, amounting to about ten per
cent of the total excise duty realised in the country. Excise duty is now
levied only on tobacco products; the duty on raw tobacco was abolished
in 1979. All manufactured products from tobacco leaf are now subject
to excise duty, with no exemption. The excise duty on cigarettes have
been progressively increased every year, so that cigarettes now provide
the major share (78 per cent) of the total excise revenue collected –
Rs. 2,488.48 crores out of Rs. 3,445.82 crores in 1994–95. The excise
duty on bidis during that year amounted to Rs. 219.91 crores, about
6.4 per cent, while those of other tobacco products (chewing, tobacco
hookah, snuff, and so on) accounted for Rs. 537.43 crores.

Significance of tobacco in India

Ever since its introduction in the 1500s, tobacco has not only got a
firm foothold in India, but has also steadily grown in importance.

India is now the third largest producer of tobacco in the world, producing 587 million kg of tobacco in 391,000 hectares of land annually.

Tobacco cultivation, processing, curing, manufacturing tobacco products, their distribution, marketing and export together constitute a major industry, employing millions of people. About 750,000 people are employed in growing, processing and curing tobacco; 20,000 in the cigarette manufacturing industries and about 3 million people in the bidi manufacturing industry. Thousands of people manufacture other tobacco products, or are employed in their distribution, marketing and exports. The bidi industry is highly labour intensive, and provides jobs for weaker sections of society, illiterate women in rural areas, and tribals.

Tobacco is a highly productive, remunerative crop to farmers. It can be grown in soils where other plants cannot be grown. The tobacco industry also provides huge profits to manufacturers and traders, and gives the government large amounts of excise duty. The foreign exchange acquired from tobacco during 1995–96 is about Rs. 421 crores.

However, there is no denying that tobacco is harmful to human kind. On an average, 60–65 per cent of Indians smoke, as compared to only 27–40 per cent of people in the West. While only 2.5 per cent of Indian women smoke, a considerably larger percentage of them chew tobacco (10 per cent).

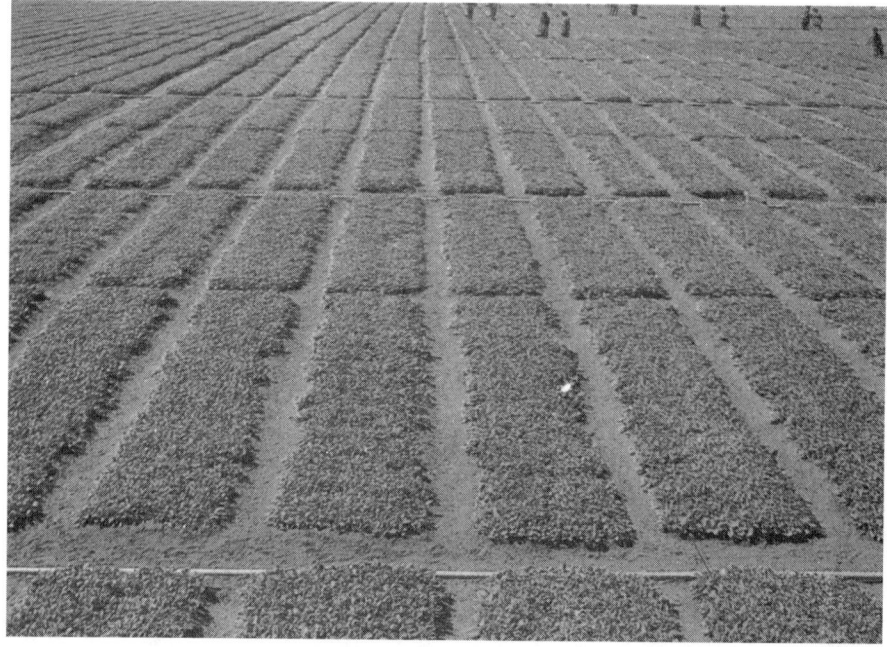

Healthy Tobacco Nursery

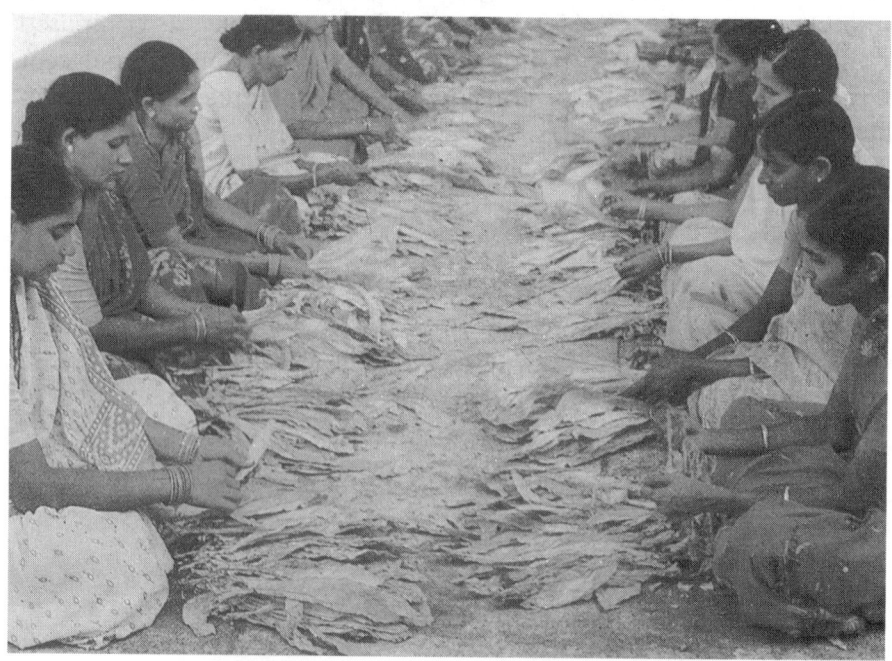

*Grading (Courtesy: M S Chari and V V Ramana,
Central Tobacco Research Institute, Rajahmundry)*

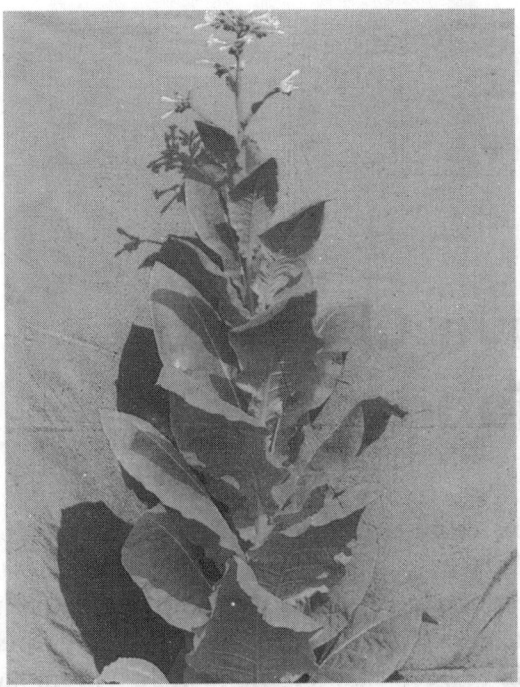

*ACR line (Courtesy: M S Chari and V V Ramana,
Central Tobacco Research Institute, Rajahmundry)*

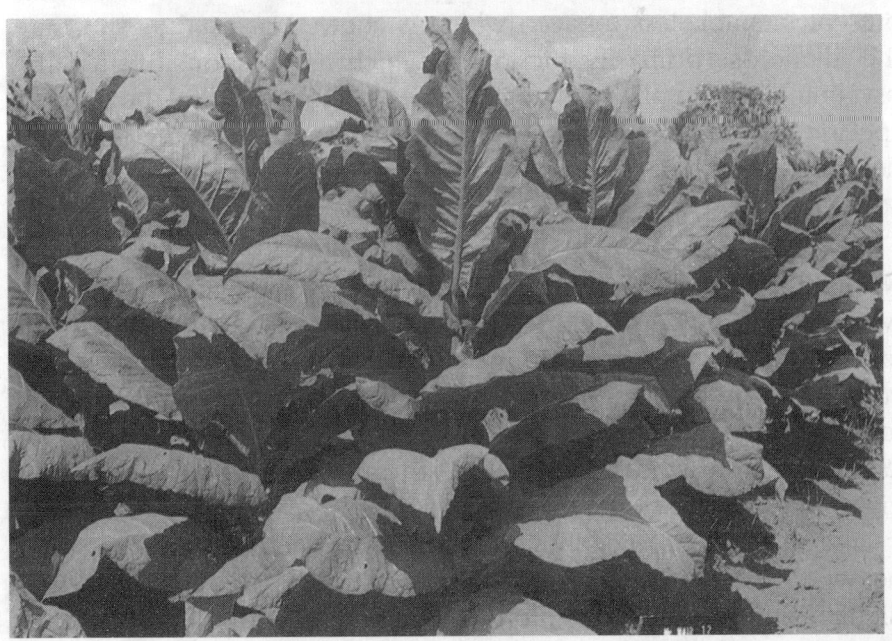

*McNair 12 (Courtesy: M S Chari and V V Ramana,
Central Tobacco Research Institute, Rajahmundry)*

6 Active Chemicals in Tobacco

Tobacco contains more than three thousand chemicals of which the most biologically active is the alkaloid, nicotine. Nicotine, which is addictive, is responsible for the physiological, psychological and pharmacological effects of tobacco. About twenty-three agents that cause tumours, have been isolated and identified in smokeless tobacco. These include the potent carcinogens, the tobacco specific N-nitrosamines. The two most important types of active chemicals present in smokeless tobacco which is chewed or used as snuff are the alkaloids (primarily nicotine), which are responsible for the psychological and pharmacological effects of tobacco, and the tobacco specific N-nitrosamines, responsible for cancer. These compounds are described below.

NICOTINE

Nicotine is a colourless, volatile liquid that gives tobacco its smell. It was isolated in 1828 from dried tobacco leaves, where it occurs to the extent of 0.5–8 per cent along with citric and malic acids. It is a colourless oily liquid, sometimes pale yellow, very hygroscopic, and turns brown when exposed to air or light. Its formula is $C_{10}H_{14}N_2$; its molecular weight is 162.23. The structure of nicotine is shown in Fig. 6.1.

Like all alkaloids, nicotine is strongly basic and miscible with water below 60 °C. It combines with almost all acids forming salts. It is highly soluble in alcohol, chloroform, ether, and other lipid solvents.

The absorption and metabolism of nicotine in the body

Free nicotine is highly lipid-soluble and hence can easily penetrate into tissues and cells, where it is readily absorbed. It exists in the free

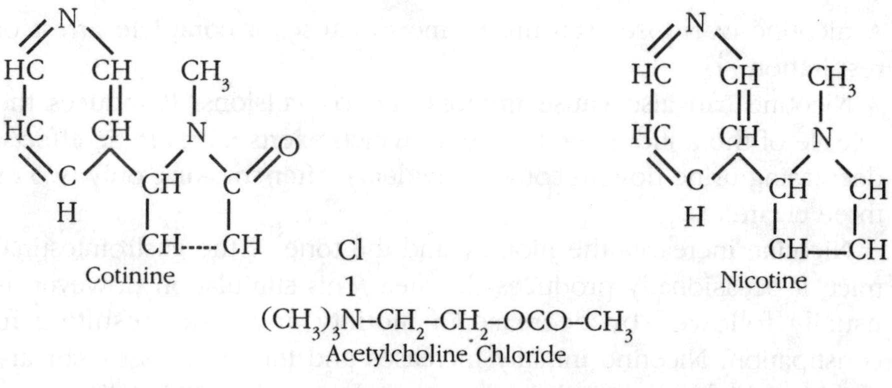

Fig. 6.1 *Structures of nicotine, cotinine and acetylcholine*

state in slightly alkaline media but as salts in acidic media. Nicotine, from chewing tobacco, cigars or pipes, is moderately absorbed in the mouth itself, by the oral mucosa. On the other hand, smoke from cigarettes, prepared from a different blend of tobacco, is slightly acidic; nicotine present in the smoke is rapidly absorbed, not so much in the mouth, but from the lungs, and hence should be inhaled, to be fully effective. The absorbed nicotine in the blood reaches and accumulates in the brain within minutes, and exerts psychological and pharmacological effects. It also enters various tissues, particularly the liver, where it is rapidly metabolised into cotinine and nicotine-N-oxide. Both these metabolites are biologically inactive. Nicotine also leaves tissues rapidly and is excreted as urine. Nicotine is so rapidly absorbed and metabolised, that cotinine appears in the blood within a few minutes of smoking. Cotinine is a useful indicator of all kinds of smoking, including passive smoking.

Nicotine absorbed from chewing tobacco, passes through the liver first, where it is partly metabolised into inactive substances, and then reaches the blood stream. It is generally less active and less harmful than the nicotine present in cigarette smoke, which is absorbed through the lungs. The latter passes directly into the blood stream, without being first inactivated in the liver. Biologically nicotine is an extremely active substance and has a wide variety of effects. It resembles the important neurotransmitter, acetylcholine in distribution of electrical charges within the molecule. Nicotine can combine with a major fraction of acetylcholine receptors (nicotinic receptors) in the body. The biological effects of nicotine are largely due to this resemblance. In low doses, it acts as a stimulating agent, just like acetylcholine, allowing impulses to pass through nerves. In larger doses, it combines with and floods all receptors, blocking the passage of all impulses. Nicotine can act as a stimulant or as a depressant, depending upon the dosage.

A nicotine overdose (60 mg or more) causes a complete arrest of respiration.

Nicotine can also cause tremors and convulsiton. It induces the release of the antidiuretic hormone, which exerts antidiuretic effects, decreasing urine flow in some individuals after smoking only two or three cigarettes.

Nicotine increases the motility and the tone of the gastrointestinal tract; it occasionally produces diarrhea. This stimulation however, is usually followed by decrease in motility and tone, resulting in constipation. Nicotine initially increases and then depresses salivary and bronchial secretion. Injecting or applying nicotine locally causes sweating, and vasoconstriction in that area.

Nicotine stimulates sympathetic ganglia and adrenal medulla, causing an increased release of catecholamines. This, in turn, results in an increase in heart rate and peripheral vasoconstriciton. Blood pressure may rise and cause an increase in the skeletal muscle and coronary blood flow.

In small doses, nicotine produces exhilaration and a feeling of well-being. It also has a soothing effect, relieving anxiety and suppressing anger. The psychological effects of nicotine, are discussed later.

Toxicity of nicotine

Nicotine is one of the most toxic agents known, and can cause death as rapidly as cyanide. Acute nicotine poisoning sometimes occurs in workers engaged in spraying nicotine (as an insecticide). Nicotine poisoning can also occur in children who accidentally consume cigarettes.

TUMOURIGENIC AGENTS

A variety of tumourigenic agents are found in natural tobacco, as well as in chewing tobacco and snuff. They include volatile aldehydes (formaldehyde, acetaldehyde, and crotonaldehyde); volatile N-nitrosamines (N-nitroso compounds of dimethylamine, pyroolidine, piperidine, morpholine and diethanolamine N-nitrosamino acids; tobacco-specific N-nitrosamines; traces of benzo(a)pyrene; nickel and cadmium; and the radioactive metals, polonium-210 and uranium-235 and   -238. Of these, the most abundant are the tobacco-specific N-nitrosamines (TSNA). They are also the most important carcinogens present in smokeless tobacco.

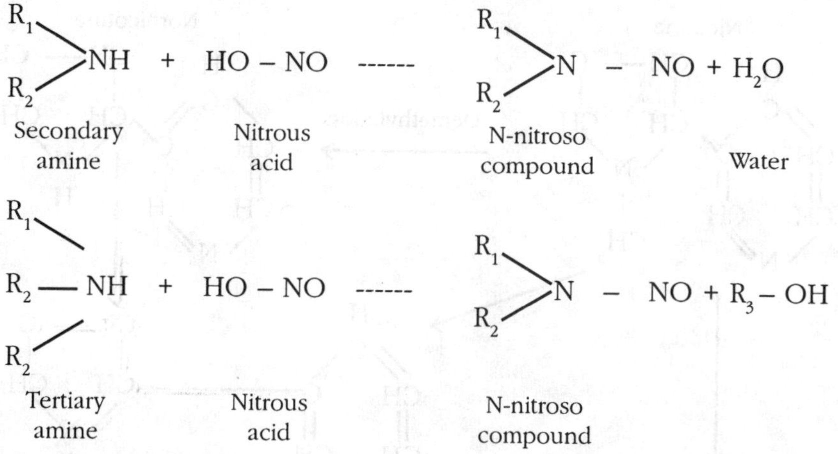

$$R_1 \diagdown NH + HO-NO \ \text{------} \ R_1 \diagup N - NO + H_2O$$

| Secondary amine | Nitrous acid | N-nitroso compound | Water |

$$R_2 - NH + HO-NO \ \text{------} \ R_1 \diagup N - NO + R_3-OH$$

| Tertiary amine | Nitrous acid | N-nitroso compound |

Fig. 6.2 *Formation of N-nitrosamines from nitrite and secondary or tertiary amines*

N-nitroso compounds are compounds containing a nitroso group, – NO, attached to a nitrogen atom in the molecule. They are usually formed by the reaction of secondary or tertiary amines with nitrous acid or nitrite in slightly acidic medium, as indicated above.

A nitrite in an acidic medium gives rise to nitrous acid. N-nitroso compounds in processed tobacco are formed by the nitrosation of precursors, present in natural tobacco during curing and fermentation. The volatile N-nitroso compounds formed from low molecular weight precursors, amount to only about one per cent of the total N-nitroso compounds. The non-volatile N-nitrosamine acids account for about 20–23 per cent. The tobacco-specific N-nitrosamines are derivatives of nicotine and other (minor) alkaloids, nornicotine, anabasine and anatabine. They constitute about 75–80 per cent of the N-nitroso compounds. Nicotine is a tertiary amine, while the other three are secondary amines. All of them yield stable nitrosamines on nitrosation. Nicotine gives rise to three potent carcinogens:

❑ N-nitrosonornicotine (NNN), which is also formed from nornicotine;

❑ 4-(N-nitrosomethylamino)-1-(3-pyridyl) butanone (NNK).

❑ 4-(N-nitrosomethylamino)-1-(3-pyridyl)-1-butanol (NNAL).

The formation of these nitrosamines are illustrated in Fig. 6.3. Of the three NNK is the most potent, producing lung cancer in all animals studied and by whichever route applied. Depending upon the species tested and mode of application, it also induces tumours in the pancreas, nasal cavity, liver, skin, and so on. NNN in drinking water when administered to rats, causes tumours in the esophagus and the nasal cavity. When injected it causes tumours of the nasal cavity alone. Swabbing the oral cavity with a mixture of NNN and

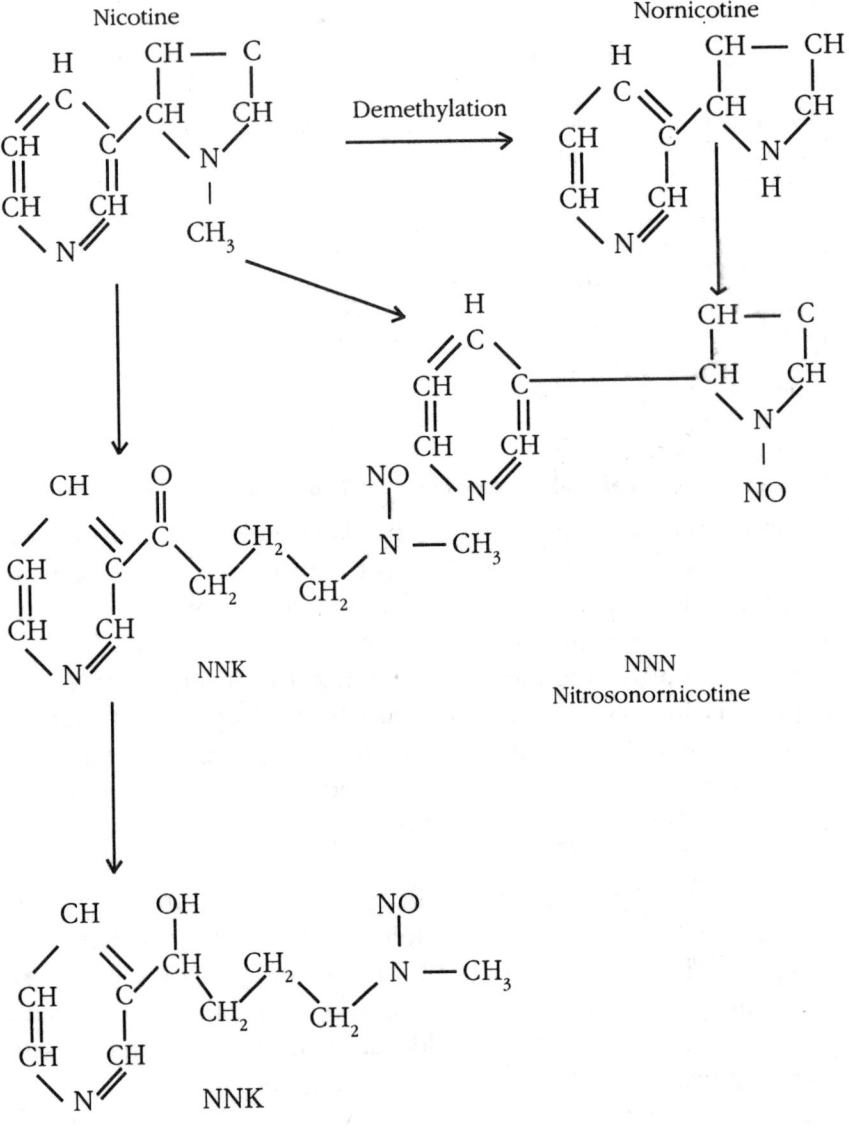

Fig. 6.3 *Formation of N-nitrosamines from tobacco alkaloids*

NNK in solution causes tumours in the oral cavity and lungs. The induction of oral cancers by NNN is considerably accelerated by the presence of HSV type 1 or HSV type 2, which act as cocarcinogens. NNAL induces tumours of the lung and pancreas in rats. N-nitrosoanatabine, NAT, is non-carcinogenic, while N-nitroso-anabasine (NAB) is weakly carcinogenic.

When one chews tobacco or uses snuff, the tobacco-specific N-nitrosamines are extracted into the saliva. There is good experimental evidence to show that endogenous nitrosation of the tobacco alkaloids takes place in the saliva itself, by using the nitrites in the saliva, and yielding more N-nitrosamines. The total TSNA ingested into the body will then be much greater than what has been actually measured from the tobacco. To a lesser extent, endogenous nitrosation can take place inside the stomach too.

The amounts of various N-nitroso compounds present in some Indian tobacco products have been measured. The preparations analysed are chewing kiwam, zarda and masheri tobaccos. The five major N-nitroso compounds present in them are NNN, NNK, NAB/NAT, N-nitroso proline (NPRO) and 3-(N-nitroso-4-methyl amino) propionic acid (NMPA). Zarda is found to contain much more of these N-nitroso compounds than others. Both moist and dry snuff used in the U.S.A. and the Scandinavian countries are found to be particularly rich in TSNAs. Snuff preparations used by Inuits (Eskimos) in Canada also contain very high amounts of TSNAs. Some types of tobacco leaves like Burley tobacco and black tobacco used in the manufacture of cigarettes in France contain large amounts of nitrates, particularly in their stems and ribs. They, in turn, give rise to higher amounts of tobacco-specific N-nitrosamine. One way of reducing the amounts of these highly carcinogenic nitrosamines would be to reduce the nitrate/nitrite content of the tobacco by suitable cultivation.

7 Active Chemicals in Tobacco Smoke

The smoke from the burning tip of cigarette, at 800 °C, is a hot mixture of many gases and particles. It is an extremely dense aerosol, with about 10^{10} particles per cubic centimeter. The particles are 0.1 to 0.50 microns in diameter. The pH of the smoke varies with the type of tobacco used. Burley or black tobacco gives rise to weakly alkaline smoke, with pH between 6.8 and 7.5. On the other hand, the smoke from flue-cured, bright tobacco, and the various blends used to make cigarettes is weakly acidic, with a pH of 5.5–6.2. The particulate matter, also known as tar, is a dark brown, sticky mass containing almost 3,500 compounds, with abundant amounts of nicotine (0.1–2.0 mg) per cigarette. If the smoke is weakly acidic, nicotine occurs primarily in the particulate phase as citrate or tartarate, but if the smoke is alkaline, it occurs as the more toxic free nicotine as both particulate and vapour.

So far, about forty-five carcinogens have been identified in cigarette smoke. They include polynuclear aromatic hydrocarbons (PAHs), with benzo(a)pyrene as the major representative of this class. They are extremely potent carcinogens, responsible for lung cancer and cancers of the upper respiratory and digestive tracts (cancers of the larynx, pharynx, mouth and esophagus). They are present in the particulate matter, that is, the tar. Catechols, also present in the tar, act as cocarcinogens, along with PAHs, and make them fully active. The tar also contains azaarenes and many aromatic amines, including the carcinogenic aromatic amines, 0-toludine (23–210 ng/cigarette), 2-naphthylamine (0.4–22 ng/cigarette) and 4-aminobiphenyl (1.3–5.0 ng/cigarette). The last two are known to cause bladder cancer in humans. Tobacco-specific N-nitrosamines, are present in smokeless tobacco and cigarette smoke. They are site-specific potent carcinogens, capable of producing tumours in the lung, trachea, nasal cavity, esophagus, pancreas, and liver. Tar also contains radioactive polonium-210, which is carcinogenic to the lungs.

Cigarette smoke also contains numerous toxic gases like carbon monoxide (CO) and hydrogen cyanide (HCN). It also contains a variety of carcinogens such as volatile N-nitrosamines, formaldehyde, benzene, acrolein, acrylonitrile, volatile phenols, and vinyl chloride. Gas in cigarette smoke can contain upto five per cent of carbon monoxide, and is higher in bidis (7.7 per cent). This is because the tendu leaf covering tobacco is not porous, unlike perforated cigarette wrappers. Carbon monoxide readily combines with the hemoglobin in the red blood cells, and prevents them from taking oxygen from the lungs to various body tissues. The affinity of carbon monoxide for hemoglobin is about two hundred times greater than that of oxygen. It forms a compound, carboxyhemoglobin which dissociates more slowly than oxyhemoglobin (oxygen and hemoglobin). The concentration of carboxyhemoglobin in the blood thus goes up with each cigarette smoked. For a heavy smoker, it can go up to as high as 15 per cent. During the night however, most of the carbon monoxide is dissociated and expelled from the lungs. As carbon monoxide is preferentially taken up from the lungs, and binds more strongly with hemoglobin than oxygen, reducing the oxygen concentration in the blood and oxygen supply to various tissues including the heart, it causes ischemia.

Carbon monoxide also adversely affects platelet aggregation and increases the cholesterol deposits in arteries. It often impairs vision, and reduces attentiveness to sound.

Hydrogen cyanide is a potent cilia toxic agent. Cilia, the fine hair-like projections inside the respiratory tract, act as filter for inhaled air, and clears the excessive secretions in the respiratory tract. Hydrogen cyanide, a compound found in cigarette smoke, prevents the cilia from performing their functions efficiently. The human body thus begins to accumulate toxic and tumourogenic agents inside the lungs, causing respiratory disorders. Rats inhaling the aldehydes in tobacco smoke, develop tumours in the nasal cavity. Benzene present in the smoke is a well-known leukemogen; smokers thus have a slightly higher risk of leukemia. The radioactive metal, polonium-210, also occurs in cigarette smoke (up to 1.0 µCi/cigarette). It is an alpha-emitter, and is found to be strongly carcinogenic, though only a minor contributor to lung cancer. Some representative tumourigenic agents present in cigarette smoke are shown in Fig. 7.1.

Tobacco smoke thus contains all the active substances that are present in smokeless tobacco particularly nicotine, potent carcinogens, and

1. Polycyclic aromatic hydrocarbon

Benzo(a)pyrene

2. Tobacco-specific nitrosamine

NNK

3. Volatile N-nitrosamine

$$CH_3 \diagdown \atop CH_3 \diagup N - N = O$$

N-Nitroso Dimethylamine

4. Aromatic amines

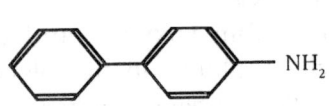

4-Aminobiphenyl

2-Naphthylamine

5. Miscellaneous organic compounds

$CH_3 - CHO$

Acetaldehyde

$CH_2 = CH - Cl$

Vinyl chloride

$CH_2 = CH - CN$

Acrilonitrile

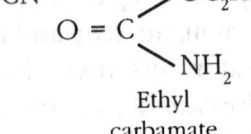

Ethyl carbamate

Benzene

6. Inorganic carcinogens

$$NH_2 - NH_2 \qquad ^{210}PO$$

Hydrazine   Polonium-210

Fig. 7.1: Some representative carcinogens present in cigarette smoke.

tobacco-specific N-nitrosamines. It also contains a large number of highly active, toxic substances formed during the combustion of tobacco in burning cigarettes. These include the reactive free radicals, the potent carcinogens, the polycyclic aromatic hydrocarbons formed as a result of pyrolysis followed by pyrosynthesis, and the toxic gases, carbon monoxide and hydrogen cyanide. Bladder carcinogens are also found in tobacco smoke. Tobacco smoke is also hot; as it passes through the respiratory system, the heat damages the respiratory tract.

All these factors make tobacco smoke infinitely more damaging than smokeless tobacco.

FILTER CIGARETTES

Realising the harmful effects of nicotine and tar, the West is now attempting to reduce their content in cigarette smoke, by using suitable blends of tobacco leaf, and introducing filter-tipped cigarettes. The outer paper covering of this cigarette is perforated, so that the inhaled smoke is diluted with air, thus reducing the carbon monoxide content. As smoke passes through the column of tobacco and the filter bed, part of the tar and the nicotine are absorbed. More than 90 per cent of cigarettes sold in the West are now filter-tipped; each cigarette yields 10–15 mg of tar, and 1.0–1.5 mg nicotine and 3.5 volume per cent of carbon monoxide. Generally, the tar and nicotine amounts in cigarettes are proportionate. In India, only half the cigarettes sold are filter-tipped; the filter length (12 mm) is only half the size of those of the west (20 mm). Indian filters are also less efficient; they are effective only to the extent of about twenty per cent as compared to about thirty per cent in the West.

Popular brands of Indian cigarettes deliver much higher levels of toxic chemicals than western cigarettes. Each Indian cigarette yields 19–28 mg of tar, 0.94–1.78 mg nicotine, and 366–638 µg hydrogen cynaide, under Standard International smoking conditions. Though bidis contain only about a fourth to a third as much tobacco as a cigarette, they yield much more toxic substances than cigarettes. This is because cigarettes are manufactured from flue-cured tobacco, while bidis are made with sun-dried, flaked tobacco. Also, while the cigarette wrapper is perforated and well-ventilated, the tendu leaf of the bidi is totally non-porous. Each bidi yields 23–41 mg tar, 1.7–2.8 mg nicotine, 7.7 volume per cent carbon monoxide and 688–904 µg hydrogen cyanide. Perforating the tendu leaf wrapper can decrease the tar and the nicotine yields but the smoke is diluted with air and hence is ineffective, leaving the smoker dissatisfied. Cotton, scented with amber, as filter in the bidi is found to be satisfactory, but has not yet become very popular. Smoking low-tar, low-nicotine cigarettes definitely reduces the risk of cancer. However, when the nicotine level becomes very low, smokers generally use more cigarettes. Recently, the U.S. government has fixed the upper limit for tar (12 mg) and nicotine (1 mg) from each cigarette.

8 Active Chemicals in the Areca Nut

The areca nut resembles tobacco in some ways. Like tobacco, it also contains many alkaloids, of which the most important is arecoline. These alkaloids like nicotine have stimulating effects on the human body. They are also probably addictive, though to a lesser degree than nicotine. The nitrosation of areca nut alkaloids yields carcinogenic N-nitrosamines, the most active among them being 3-(methyl-nitrosamino)-propionitrile (MNPN).

Areca nut preparations are as widely used in India as tobacco products and can have harmful long-term biological effects. While tobacco and snuff cause oral cancers and leukoplakia, a person who habitually chews the areca nut is susceptible to leukoplakia, and the more serious submucous fibrosis. Like tobacco, areca nut also occupies a significant position in the Indian economy. The areca palm is grown in about 184,500 hectares in India, and produces about 191,400 tonnes of nuts every year. This chapter explores some details about the areca nut, areca nut alkaloids, and the nitrosamines formed by them.

The areca palm (*Areca catechu L.*) belongs to the family of Palmaceae. It is cultivated mainly in India and the East Indies. The fruit of the areca nut is orange-yellow (Fig. 8.1). The dried nut is a heavy, brown, mottled structure that is rounded and depressed at the base. On the outside, it is brown, mottled with fawn. The inside of the areca nut is brown-red and has white veins. When chewed, the thin slices of the nut taste pungent. The fresh fruits have a faint cheese-like odour. Processed areca nut preparations like supari (scented betel nut) use various additives and sweetening and flavouring agents.

The areca nut is composed of carbohydrates (50–75 per cent), fats (14 per cent), proteins (5–8 per cent), red tannins (15 per cent), lkaloids, and other nitrogenous bases such as choline.

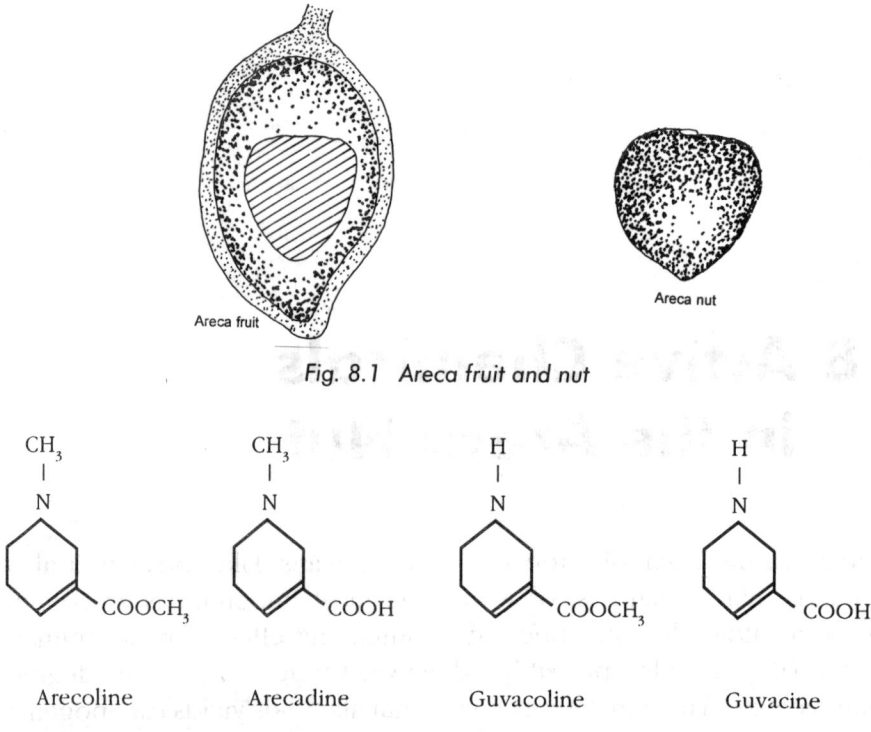

Fig. 8.1   Areca fruit and nut

Fig. 8.2   Areca nut alkaloids

Alkaloids in the areca nut

The alkaloids present in areca nut are the structurally related compounds arecoline, arecaidine, guvacine, and guvacoline (Fig. 8.2). Arecaidine and guvacoline are isomers, containing one methyl group less than arecoline. Both the methyl groups of arecoine are absent in guvacine. Among these alkaloids, arecoline is by far the most important, occurring to the extent of 0.5–0.7 per cent in areca nut. Its molecular formula is $C_8H_{13}NO_2$, and molecular weight is 155.19. Arecoline is an oily liquid, with a boiling point of 209 °C and a strong base, which is freely miscible with water, alcohol and ether. Arecoline mimics the action of acetylcholine, and stimulates both the central and the peripheral nervous system. The emphoric effect of areca nut is due to arecotine. Nitrosation of these alkaloids takes place in the mouth through the nitrites in the saliva. Nitrosation of arecoline, the major alkaloid in betel nut and betel quid, yields four N-nitroso compounds (Fig. 8.3) N-nitrosoguvacoline (NG), N-nitrosoguvacine (NGC), 3-(methyl-nitrosamino) propionitrile (MNPN); and 3-(methylnitrosamino) propionaldehyde (MNPA). Among these N-nitroso compounds, MNPN is highly genotoxic, and is a carcinogen, inducing benign and malignant tumours in the esophagus, the tongue, the nasal cavity, and the liver

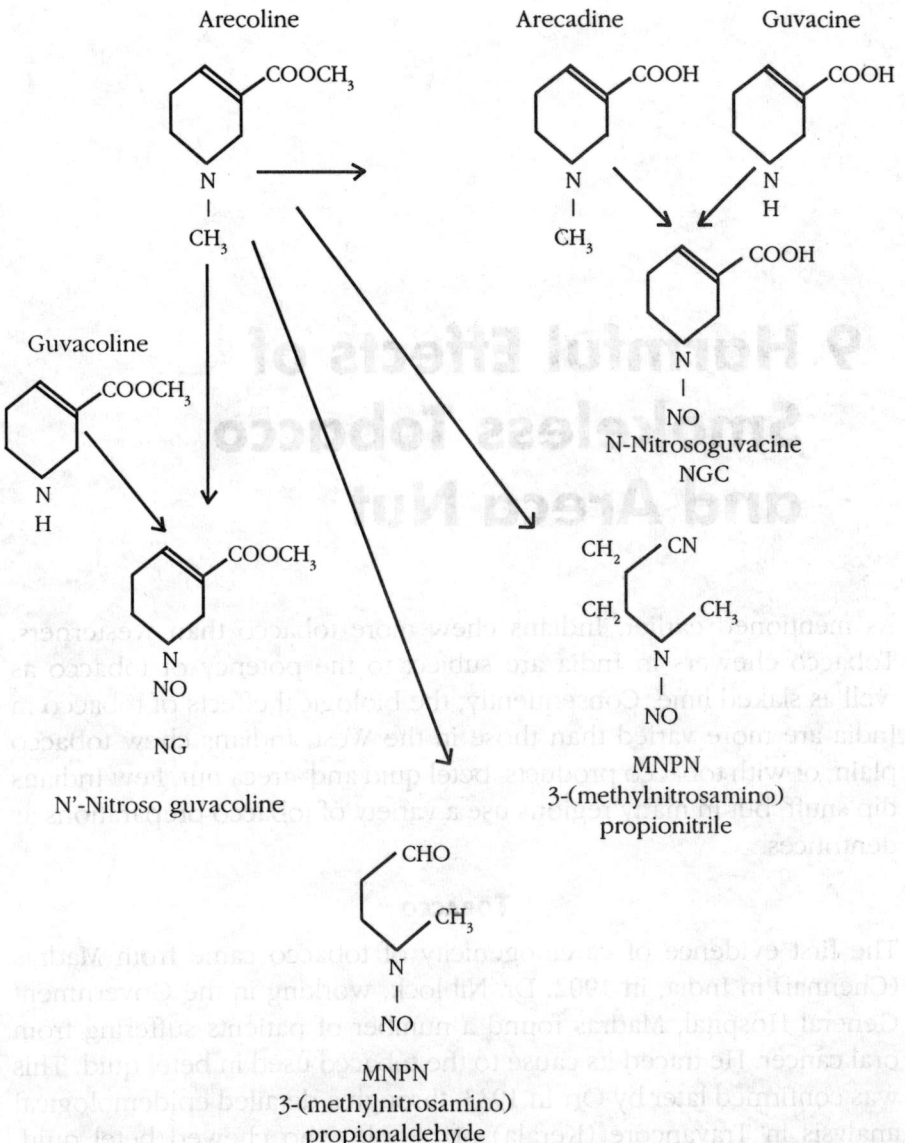

Fig. 8.3 N-nitrosamine derived from areca nut alkaloids

of the F344 rats. NG induces tumours of the exocrine pancreas in these rats. MNPA is highly genotoxic. NGC has not been investigated so far.

9 Harmful Effects of Smokeless Tobacco and Areca Nut

As mentioned earlier, Indians chew more tobacco than westerners. Tobacco chewers in India are subject to the potency of tobacco as well as slaked lime. Consequently, the biological effects of tobacco in India are more varied than those in the West. Indians chew tobacco plain, or with tobacco products, betel quid and areca nut. Few Indians dip snuff, but in many regions use a variety of tobacco preparations as dentrifices.

Tobacco

The first evidence of carcinogenicity of tobacco came from Madras (Chennai) in India, in 1902. Dr. Niblock, working in the Government General Hospital, Madras found a number of patients suffering from oral cancer. He traced its cause to the tobacco used in betel quid. This was confirmed later by Orr in 1933, through a detailed epidemological analysis in Travancore (Kerala) of people who chewed betel quid. A number of investigations have been conducted since then on the carcinogenicity of tobacco, betel quid, and various components of betel quid. The results reveal that tobacco, whether chewed alone, with betel quid, with lime, as khaini, or with lime and the areca nut, as Mainpuri tobacco, is carcinogenic. It causes cancer particularly in those locations, which have been in close contact with tobacco for a long time – the buccal mucosa, the gum or the mandibular groove, or the tongue. In some states like Bihar and Uttar Pradesh, a mixture of tobacco and slaked lime, is often placed in the lower labial groove and held against the labial mucosa. This causes cancer of the lower labial mucosa (the inner surface of the lip) in due course. This is the area most frequently affected by cancer. In places where people chew betel quid, up to 80 per cent of oral cancers occur in the left buccal mucosa, rather than in the right. This is perhaps due to the tendency to keep the betel quid on the left side of the mouth. The carcinogenicity of smokeless tobacco is further confirmed by the fact that snuff dipping in the West causes oral cancer just where the pinch of snuff is placed. The carcinogens involved here are tobacco-specific nitrosamines. Epidemiological research carried out in Uttar Pradesh has shown that chewing Mainpuri tobacco leads to oral cancer, which is aggravated by simultaneous smoking, and still further by drinking alcohol. Oral cancer was highest among men, (11.2 per 1,000), who chewed Mainpuri tobacco, smoked, and drank alcohol. Chewing tobacco can also cause the pre-cancerous lesion, leukoplakia, characterised by white patches on the tongue or the buccal mucosa.

BETEL QUID

Whether or not betel quid by itself is carcinogenic, is uncertain. Case-control studies in Sri Lanka revealed that chewing betel quid without tobacco carries an insignificant risk for oral cancer. Betel leaves (Piper betel), by themselves, are known to prevent carcinogenesis. They contain volatile oils such as eugenol and terpenes, nitrates, small quantities of sugar, starch, tannin, and several other substances. Epidemiological investigations have shown that while betel quid, without tobacco contributes insignificantly to oral cancer, it leads to oral and pharyngeal cancers when accompanied by smoking. Smoking and chewing betel quid with tobacco, causes oropharyngeal and hypopharyngeal cancers, rather than oral cancer.

ARECA NUT

While endogenous nitrosation of areca nut alkaloids can give rise to carcinogenic nitrosamines, it is not known if, and to what extent, this occurs inside the body. We need to investigate the contribution of various areca nut preparations to oral and pharyngeal cancers. The Assamese chew an areca nut preparation known as taamool, or bura taamool, but it is not known whether this is responsible for the high incidence of pharyngeal cancers among them. Habitually chewing the areca nut alone, as supari, as betel quid, with lime, tobacco, or with sweetening and flavouring agents such as paan masala, definitely causes two important pre-cancers, the pre-cancerous lesion leukoplakia, and the pre-cancerous condition, submucous fibrosis (SMF).

Leukoplakia

Leukoplakia is the most common precancerous lesion, occurring as a white patch or plaque, anywhere in the oral cavity. The incidence of leukoplakia varies from 0.2–4.9 per cent in India. According to the World Health Organization (W.H.O.) leukoplakia is "a raised white patch of the oral mucosa measuring five millimeters or more, which cannot be scraped off, and which cannot be attributed to any other diagnosable disease". Leukoplakias may occur as three types: 84 per cent as homogeneous leukoplakias, where the lesions are predominantly white, though greyish or yellowish patches can also occur; upto 13 per cent as ulcerated leukoplakia, which are reddish areas with or without yellowish fibrin or white patches; and 3 per cent as nodular leukoplakia, also called *speckled leukoplakia*, characterised by small white specks or nodules on an erythematous base. Leukoplakia is essentially a reversible condition. It can persist for a long time, regress spontaneously and recur, or progress to cancer. The leukoplakia will regress faster if one stops chewing suspected carcinogens. About 3–6 per cent of all leukoplakias may become malignant. Nodular leukoplakias exhibit greater dysplasia, have greater malignant potential with about a fifth progressing to cancer. Some changes, which occur during this transformation to early oral cancer, are development of thick/nodular areas, ulcers, rolled margins, growths, or indurated areas.

Submucous fibrosis

Oral submucous fibrosis is the more serious pre-cancerous condition. It occurs predominantly among resident and non-resident Indians. It occurs to a lesser extent among other Asians, and only occasionally among Europeans. Submucous fibrosis occurs primarily due to chewing areca nut and probably due to eating chillies too. Submucous fibrosis occurs in about 3.8 million Indians (0.4 per cent of the population). This number is increasing rapidly thanks to greater consumption of various areca nut preparations like pan masala, and mawa. Submucous fibrosis is a chronic mucosa condition, characterised by a mucosal rigidity of varying intensity. It can occur in any part of the oral mucosa. This rigidity is due to the fibroelastic transformation of the underlying connective tissue. Submucous fibrosis is diagnosed by the presence of palpable fibrous bands, which can occur in the buccal mucosa, retromolar area and around the rim oris. If the tongue is affected, it becomes depapillated and very smooth. Because it gradually becomes rigid, the tongue progressively loses its mobility and ability to protrude.

In severe cases, the patient will experience considerable difficulty in opening his mouth. The most common symptom of submucosa fibrosis, is a burning sensation of the oral mucosa, which is aggravated by spicy food. Hypersalivation or dryness of the mouth can occur. A common trait of submucous fibrosis is *blanching*, a white, marble-like appearance of the oral mucosa. Blanching occurs due to impairment of local vascularity. The disease often starts as a blanched area, and then developes palpable fibrous bands. The incubation period for submucous fibrosis (the time taken for the disease to develop) ranges from a few months to several decades. People chewing areca nut alone supari have a considerably shorter incubation period than those chewing betel quid.

Among Indians SMF occurs in the buccal mucosa in about 98 per cent. The affected mucosa initially becomes coarse, tough, and leathery, developing vertical fibrous bands as the disease progresses. Submucous fibrosis of the tongue and the floor of the mouth occur to a greater extent in Ernakulam (Kerala) than in Bhavnagar (Gujarat) where there is a greater incidence of submucous fibrosis of the soft palate and uvula. These differences are probably due to the types of areca nut preparations chewed at these places, and the way in which they are chewed.

Unlike leukoplakia, SMF is not known to regress either spontaneously, or when the person stops chewing the areca nut. The condition may remain unchanged or become severe, involving additional areas of the oral mucosa. In this condition, the epithelium is atrophic and highly susceptible to carcinogens. Thus, about 7–8 per cent of cases of submucous fibrosis develop into oral cancers. Submucous fibrosis coexisting with leukoplakia stands an even greater risk of being transformed into malignant oral cancer. While surgery and therapy can relieve severe symptoms of submucous fibrosis and open the mouth, there is no definitive treatment yet to completely restore the oral mucosa.

Oral cancer

The term oral cancer is used to describe any malignancy that arises from the oral mucosa in the mouth. Histologically, squamous cell carcinoma is the most common type of oral cancer, representing 90–95 per cent of all oral malignancies. In the International Classification of Diseases, published by the W.H.O., (ICD-9) the code numbers 140 (lip), 141 (tongue), 142 (salivary glands), 143 (gingiva), 144 (floor of the mouth), and 145 (other parts of the mouth) are assigned to cancers at the intra-oral sites indicated. Oral cancer is among the ten most common cancers in the world. In India, it constitutes about a tenth of all cancers, ranking from first to sixth most common cancer in different regions. The most common sites at which oral cancers occur in our country are the tongue (anterior two-thirds) and the buccal mucosa. Chewing tobacco alone or with betel quid, is the primary cause of oral cancers, followed by smoking. According to the W.H.O., almost ninety per cent of all oral cancers are due to tobacco. Areca nut causes two pre-cancers, leukoplakia and submucous fibrosis, and through them, a very small percentage of oral cancers too.

Oral cancer, leukoplakia and submucous fibrosis are the primary ill effects of smokeless tobacco. These tobacco chewing habits are responsible for the high rates of oral cancer in India. Among women, the highest incidence of oral cancer in the whole world, occurs in Bangalore.

Other effects of chewing

Chewing betel quid increases salivation, decreases the sense of taste, and alters sensory perceptions of the buccal mucosal tissues. It increases the occurrence of periodontal disease and decreases the occurence of caries. It also imparts a bright red colour to the oral mucosa. The colour is transient in occasional chewers, but permanently stains the mucosa of habitual and heavy chewers. The bright red colour produced is caused by 0-quinone from the water-soluble polyphenols, notably leucocynidins, at the alkaline pH of 8.9 through secondary reactions. The colour can usually be washed off by repeatedly rinsing one's mouth. Habitual betel quid chewing can produce black stains on the teeth. The stain has a composition similar to that of calculus, and probably protects the teeth against caries. Habitual chewing also produces thick brown-black encrustations where the betel quid is placed. The encrustation can be scraped off with a piece of gauze, and does not lead to leukoplakia. Chewing betel quid also causes other mucosal changes, such as dryness of the mucosa, focal erosion, ulceration and atrophy of the tongue mucosa.

A notable effect of oral tobacco usage is gingival recession, where the tobacco, snuff, or khaini, has been placed and held against the gum. Often, a well-defined, thick, yellowish white plaque is also produced in the groove, where the khaini is held. It is very similar to the betel quid encrustation among heavy paan chewers, and can be scraped off with gauze. In Maharashtra, this lesion is found much more frequently (in 2.9 per cent) than leukoplakia (in 0.6 per cent).

SNUFF AND DENTIFRICES

Dipping snuff in India is not as common as in the West, inhaling being a practice more or less only in Tamil Nadu and West Bengal. The biological effects of snuff and other dentifrices like mishri (masheri), bajjar and gudhaku, have not been studied in detail. Among these, mishri, which is pyrolised tobacco powder, contains potent carcinogens, like polycyclic aromatic hydrocarbons, in addition to tobacco-specific nitrosamines. While all these tobacco preparations are stimulatory, addictive, and carcinogenic, we still do not know how hazardous they actually are. A thorough investigation of their effects needs to be carried out.

10 Harmful Effects of Smoking: COLD and Shorter Life Span

Cigarette smoke is a unique mixture of highly reactive potent toxins, which seriously damage the body affecting both the respiratory and vascular systems, and inducing malignant tumours in the respiratory, digestive, and urinary tracts. While its ability to induce a fatal lung cancer is well-known, the public is not fully aware of its other equally damaging effects: shortening life spans, chronic obstructive lung disease (COLD), ischemic heart disease (IHD) and myocardial infarction (MI).

SHORTER LIFE SPAN

One of the earliest recorded damaging effects of smoking is a shortening of life span. In 1938, Professor Raymond Pearl of the Johns Hopkins University provided statistical evidence that non-smokers live longer than smokers. He showed that 67 per cent of non-smokers lived for over sixty years, as against 46 per cent of smokers, at that time. Smoking tobacco is now generally accepted as the most important cause of premature death, and the cause of chronic ill health, in most industrialised countries. About a fifth of all deaths in developed countries is due to smoking.

It has been estimated by Sanghvi, Jayant, and Notani, of the Tata Memorial Centre, Mumbai, in 1986 that in India alone, smoking was responsible for 9.86 million cases of chronic obstructive lung disease (of which 157,000 patients died), 1.27 million cases of coronary heart disease (of which 101,000 patients died), 27,000 deaths due to the cerebrovascular disease, and 270,000 cases of cancer in the upper alimentary and respiratory tracts (of which 69,000 patients died). Smoking is undoubtedly the most important single, preventable cause of illness, a fact that is now acknowledged by 70 per cent of smokers.

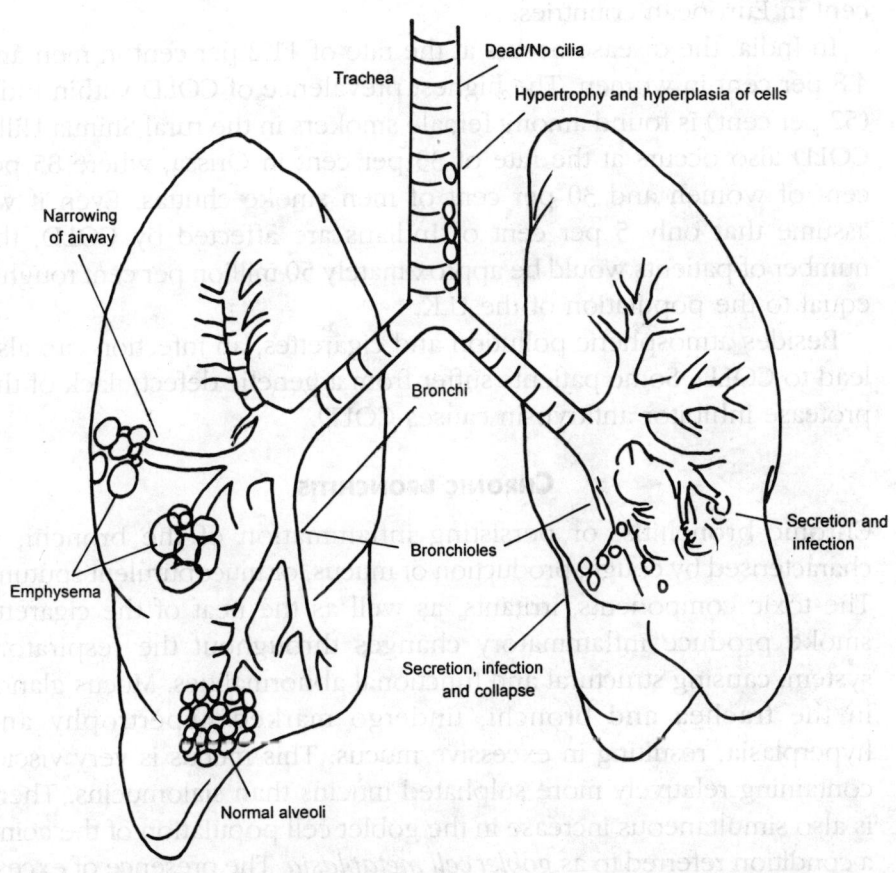

Dead/No cilia

Trachea

Hypertrophy and hyperplasia of cells

Narrowing
of airway

Bronchi

Secretion and
infection

Bronchioles

Emphysema

Secretion, infection
and collapse

Normal alveoli

*Fig. 10.1   Changes in the lungs of a heavy smoker: a bunch of
normal alveoli are shown for comparison*

Chronic Obstructive Lung Disease

Both cigarette and bidi smoking cause chronic obstructive lung disease,
also known as chronic obstructive airways disease (COAD). Chronic
obstructive airways disease has two major components: chronic
bronchitis and emphysema. They can exist separately, but often occur
together. It is difficult to differentiate them clinically. COLD also causes
a thickening and narrowing of airways, and obstructs the respiratory
flow. Atmospheric pollution is the main cause of these diseases and

the most significant polluting agent is cigarette smoke. These diseases are more common in industrialised societies, chronic obstructive lung disease being the fifth common cause of death in the U.S.A. Its prevalence varies from 11.2–32.8 per cent in the U.K, and 9–28 per cent in European countries.

In India, the disease occurs at the rate of 11.2 per cent in men and 4.8 per cent in women. The highest prevalence of COLD within India (52 per cent) is found among female smokers in the rural Shimla Hills. COLD also occurs at the rate of 33 per cent in Orissa, where 85 per cent of women and 30 per cent of men smoke chuttas. Even if we assume that only 5 per cent of Indians are affected by COLD, the number of patients would be approximately 50 million per cent roughly equal to the population of the U.K.

Besides atmospheric pollution and cigarettes, an infection can also lead to COLD. Some patients suffer from a genetic defect, lack of the protease inhibitor antitrypsin causes COLD.

CHRONIC BRONCHITIS

Chronic bronchitis, or persisting inflammation of the bronchi, is characterised by cough, production of mucus, or mucopurulent sputum. The toxic components, irritants, as well as the heat of the cigarette smoke produce inflammatory changes throughout the respiratory system, causing structural and functional abnormalities. Mucus glands in the trachea and bronchi, undergo marked hypertrophy and hyperplasia, resulting in excessive mucus. This mucus is very viscid, containing relatively more sulphated mucins than sialomucins. There is also simultaneous increase in the goblet cell population of the acini, a condition referred to as *goblet cell metaplasia*. The presence of excess intraluminal mucus within the bronchioles prevents air from passing through. Hydrogen cyanide present in cigarette smoke is a very powerful ciliary toxin, which deactivates the mucociliary clearance system. The excessive mucus produced thus remains uncleared, and stagnates in the body. This in turn blocks the air passages, and permanently damages certain areas of the lungs. Particles inhaled from the cigarette remain in the lungs, injuring the lung tissues. The patient, in attempting to clear his lungs, coughs violently, and brings out a large amount of viscid phlegm – typical symptoms of bronchitis. The smaller, peripheral, airways narrow because they are attached to the interlobular septa of the lungs.

Smoking also thickens and narrows small airways in the lungs. Both the lumen and the wall of the air passage become inflamed, and begin accumulating mucus. The bronchiolar wall then develop edema. The smooth muscle undergoes hypertrophy, resulting in an increase in tone and reactivity. Peribronchiolar fibrosis also occurs, leading to a loss of tethering of the small airways in the surrounding intralobular septa of the lungs. This results in a bronchiolar narrowing during expiration, and obstructs the flow of air inside the lungs.

The elastic recoil of the lung tissue pushes out air from the lungs during expiration. Smoking interferes with this function by decreasing the elastic recoil of the lung tissue, and hence the volume of air expired. The forced expiratory volume per second (FEV$_1$) which is a good indicator of lung function, is progressively reduced in smokers.

EMPHYSEMA

Emphysema is defined as permanent over-distension of the air passages distal to the terminal bronchioles, associated with destruction of the walls of air spaces (alveoli) within the acini. The walls of the alveoli (tiny air sacs within the lungs) begin to break down, thus reducing the surface area of the lungs. The hemoglobin in the circulating blood begins to absorb less oxygen from the lungs. The changes in the lungs following smoking are illustrated in Figs. 10.1 and 10.2.

The destruction of the alveolar walls is brought about by the enzymes, collagenase and elastase, released from neutrophils and macrophages inside the lungs. The alveolar walls are composed of the proteins, collagen types I and II, elastin, proteoglycans and fibronectin. Under normal circumstances, the alveolar walls and other connective tissue in the lungs remain intact because of the framework of the lung parenchyma, which is preserved by the presence of the protease inhibitor α-antitrypsin. Alpha-antitrypsin is a glycoprotein with methionine at its active site. It binds to the proteolytic enzymes through methionine, and inhibits their functioning. Cigarette smoke, with its rich content of free radicals and other toxins, upsets this balance in two ways, and destroys the alveolar walls. It activates the neutrophils and macrophages, causing them to release their intralysosomal enzymes, collagenase and elastase. Simultaneously, it inactivates α-antitrypsin by oxidation at the active site, leaving the proteolytic enzymes, collagenase and elastase, free to act. The large reduction in total lung surface caused by partial destruction of the alveolar walls, seriously hampers the gaseous exchange between the oxygen in the air and the carbon dioxide in the circulating blood that occurs at these surfaces. The patient often struggles to get enough oxygen into his system.

Emphysema commonly occurs in older people, in the upper parts of the lung. But it can occur in people below forty, if they are deficient

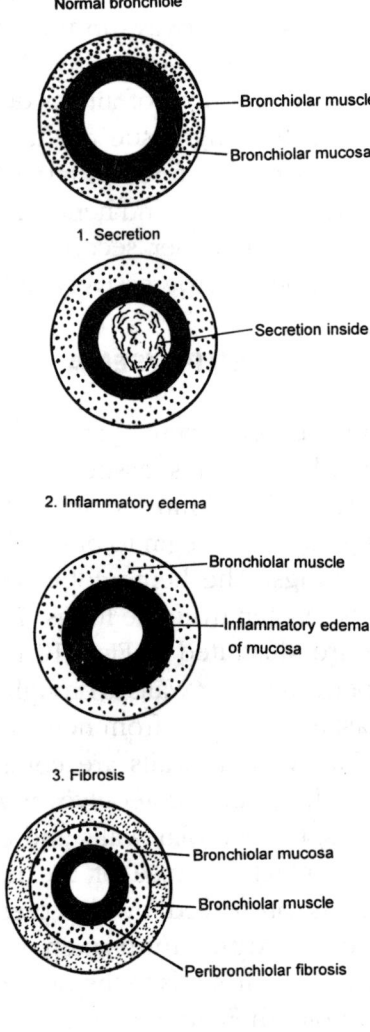

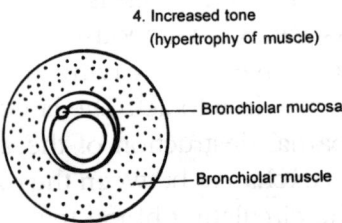

Fig. 10.2   Narrowing of the airways following smoking

in the enzyme inhibitor α-antitrypsin. Computed tomography helps localise and assess the severity of the emphysematous areas within the lungs.

The free radicals in cigarette smoke cause peroxidation of the membrane lipids, thus altering the permeability of the bronchial epithelium.

Chronic obstructive airways disease progresses slowly, and is accompanied by gradual loss of lung function. Patients can live with it for years and then die with it, rather than because of it. However, it can cripple a person's life and lead to premature death, by severely depressing lung function. The mortality to morbidity ratio in COLD is only 1.6 per cent.

Dust can also cause COLD. Many of our cities are dusty and highly polluted. A clean environment where people avoid smoking, will go a long way in the prevention of respiratory disorders in our country.

11 Harmful Effects of Smoking: Cardiovascular Diseases

In the West, cardiovascular diseases rank as the number one killer. They are responsible for about 27 per cent of all deaths in Britain. The most important contributing factor to cardiovascular diseases is found to be cigarette smoking, which causes about forty per cent of all deaths from cardiovascular diseases. Epidemiological studies reveal that there is a strong positive correlation between smoking more than fifteen cigarettes per day, and the risk of ischemic heart disease (IHD), stroke and peripheral arterial insufficiency. Further, it has been shown that a decrease in smoking results in a significant decrease in premature death due to coronary heart disease. Epidemiological studies carried out by various groups in the U.S.A., Japan, Sweden, Finland and other countries confirm that cigarette smoke is the chief cause of cardiovascular diseases.

ISCHEMIA

The energy requirements of the heart are very high. The heart muscles need energy to maintain their periodic contractions, and the integrity of their membranes, and the Na^+, K^+ and Ca^{++} concentration gradients. The heart is highly vascularised, and meets its energy requirements by oxidising glucose and free fatty acids in the blood. However, if the blood flow in the coronary vessels is impeded, the heart's energy requirements will not be met and it has to use glycogen, its poor energy reserve. The heart, thus cannot survive for more than a few minutes if the blood supply to its muscle is blocked, as happens in coronary thrombosis.

The brain is an equally sensitive organ. It can utilise only glucose as its metabolic fuel to meet all its energy requirements. It cannot survive without oxygen for more than three to four minutes. Both the heart and the brain get their oxygen and other nutritional requirements only through blood circulation. If the blood supply to the brain through the carotid arteries is blocked, there will be an immediate loss of consciousness, and the nerve cells in the brain, the neurons, will begin to die after three or four minutes.

Similarly, if the blood supply to a particular region of the heart is cut off by a block in the corresponding coronary artery, the heart muscle cells there will undergo necrosis and die, creating an area of dead tissue; this is termed *myocardial infarction.* Unfortunately, neither neurons nor heart muscle cells can regenerate themselves, so once affected the damage is permanent.

The three most important processes involved in blocking blood vessels are atherosclerosis, thrombosis, and embolism. Smoking promotes both atherosclerosis and thrombosis. The components of cigarette smoke can also induce ischaemia of the heart, where the heart's oxygen supply is far below its metabolic requirements, due to low perfusion. The results can be catastrophic. The on going Framingham prospective study mentions that cigarette smoking causes sudden coronary death and acute myocardial infarction. Nicotine and carbon monoxide are the two most important constituents of cigarette smoke responsible for this; however other constituents like hydrogen cyanide, oxides of nitrogen and carbon disulphide also contribute to coronary diseases.

Atherosclerosis

Atherosclerosis is a disorder characterised by deposition of fibrolipids in arteries. It is confined to large, elastic and muscular arteries with a diameter of more than 300 μm such as the aorta, epicardial coronary, femoral, and carotid arteries. Fibrolipids deposit predominantly in the intimal layer of the vessel wall. The deposit, called plaque, originates from monocytes adhering to the endothelium of the blood vessel, then getting into the intima and accumulating lipids inside, and transforming into macrophage foamy cells. Larger amounts of extracellular lipids are concentrated inside. The deposit also contains fibrin strands produced by smooth muscle cells. Atherosclerosis in early stages is asymptomatic, characterised by small patches of fibrolipids in blood vessels. At this stage, it is composed mainly of macrophage foamy cells containing lipids and fibrin strands. Fatty dots or streaks are observed. Advanced plaque is formed by the action of platelets and of fibrinogen. When platelets come into contact with the blood vessel wall, they are activated, releasing pro-aggregatory factors like thromboxane A_2 and adenosine diphosphate (ADP). The platelets then begin to aggregate by adhering to each other, forming a mass of activated cells. Fibrinogen bridges are formed between adjacent platelets. More and more platelets are activated, and begin to accumulate. Advanced atherosclerotic plaques contain a mass of platelets and fibrin over a lipid core. Deep inside the plaque, the lipid core is seen as a soft, yellow, semi-fluid mass. It is covered by a collageneous matrix-rich connective tissue called a cap, which lies just under the endothelium (Fig. 11.1). The composition of the atheromatous plaque can vary widely. Lipid-rich plaques are yellow while plaques that primarily contain fibrin are white. These plaques narrow the lumen of the blood vessel. This process is known as stenosis; it seriously impedes the smooth flow of blood.

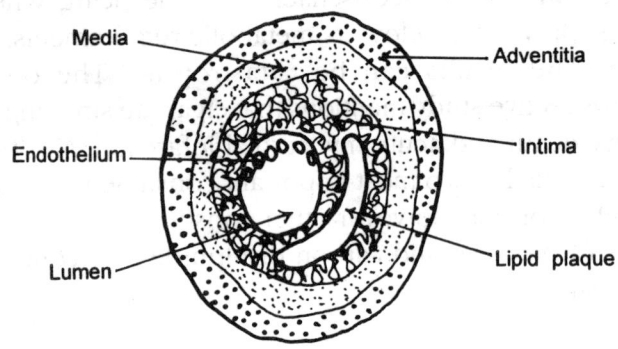

Fig.11.1   Atheromatous plaque

Thrombosis

Thrombosis is a complication arising out of atherosclerosis. A thrombus is defined as a solid mass or plug formed within the heart, arteries, veins or capillaries, from the components of the streaming blood. Thrombosis is the process of forming a thrombus, and subsequent blocking of an artery. It involves the adhesion of platelets over an abnormal vascular surface, and aggregation to form a plug, which blocks the artery. Aggregates of platelets deposited over an atheromatous plaque can also peel off as a small mass, travel in the blood stream, and cause thrombosis, where the blood vessel becomes too narrow for it to pass through. Partial blocking of an artery results in underperfusion of the tissue served by it, and consequent ischemia. However, complete blocking or the occlusion of an artery, will have far more serious consequences like myocardial infarction, sudden coronary death, complete loss of consciousness and so on. The term embolism refers to complete blocking of a blood vessel by an agent, including foreign substances. Ninety per cent of embolism occurs due to occlusion by thrombi.

The role of smoking

Smoking promotes ischemia, atherosclerosis, and thrombosis in a variety of ways. Nicotine induces the release of catecholamines, which increase the heart and pulse rates, and oxygen consumption by the heart muscle. Simultaneously, the carbon monoxide present in cigarette smoke, combines with hemoglobin in blood cells forming carboxyhemoglobin, and decreases the oxygen transport and supply to various tissues, including the heart. Thus, smoking increases the heart muscles' demand for oxygen while decreasing oxygen availability. It creates an ischemia of the heart, which is responsible for 60 per cent of sudden coronary deaths. Both nicotine and carbon monoxide promote platelet aggregation, a key factor causing thrombosis. Catecholamines also increase the systolic pressure, the levels of free fatty acids, and the level of blood sugar, all of which are associated with ischemic heart disease. Carbon monoxide increases the deposition of cholesterol in blood vessels, promoting atherosclerosis, which is found to be more extensive and severe in smokers than in non-smokers.

Cigarette smoking is known to cause changes in platelet functions and clotting parameters. A commonly found effect of smoking is a significant increase in the levels of plasma fibrinogen, which can cause ischemic heart diseases, and strokes. High levels of plasma fibrinogen also causes thrombosis in a variety of ways. The viscosities of plasma as well as of whole blood are markedly increased, thus favouring the onset of thrombosis.

Plasma fibrinogen enhances platelet aggregation. In animals exposed to fresh cigarette smoke, platelets are found to adhere to intact endothelium. Cigarette smoke also markedly reduces the production of prostacyclin, which inhibits platelet aggregation.

Cigarette smoking markedly decreases fibrinolytic activity. Fibrinolysis enhances the enzymatic breakdown of fibrin into simpler compounds. This facilitates the removal of fibrin from atheromatous deposits and thrombi, and reduces the risk from death. Cigarette smoking acts as an inhibitor to this process leading to thrombosis and ischemic heart diseases. Thus, smoking actively contributes to ischemic heart diseases such as myocardial infarction and sudden coronary death in both men and women.

Carbon monoxide in cigarette smoke, has other debilitating effects. It impairs vision, and reduces judgement and attentiveness. Heavy smoking is thus very harmful to automobile drivers and pilots. As carbon monoxide adversely affects oxygen transport to various tissues, including muscles, smoking will also seriously reduce athletic performance.

12 Harmful Effects of Smoking: Malignancy

It was lung cancer, which brought to light the harmful effects of smoking during the 1960s. Though smoking causes chronic obstructive lung disease only a small percentage of people die of it. On the other hand, lung cancer is fatal. Only 10–15 per cent of lung cancer patients survive for one year after diagnosis, and the five-year survival rate is about 7–10 per cent. Smoking leads to more cases of coronary heart disease than cancer, but is only one of the causes of coronary heart disease, the other causes being hypertension, hyperlipidemia, diabetes and obesity. On the other hand, lung cancer is almost exclusively due to smoking. About 85–90 per cent of lung cancer patients have been found to be either current or ex-smokers.

The correlation between smoking and the incidence of lung cancer was established by the pioneering investigations of Doll and Hill in the U.K., and Hammond and co-workers in the U.S.A, in the late 1950s. Working with 40,637 British male doctors, Doll and Hill showed that the risk of developing lung cancer in men, who smoked more than twenty-five cigarettes a day, was 25 times that of non-smokers. A similar conclusion was reached by Hammond and Horn, who studied the consequences of smoking in 187,873 men in the U.S.A. Detailed investigations by Wynder and the co-workers in the U.S.A. over a number of years, later supported these findings. Since then, thirty retrospective studies and eight prospective studies in many countries all over the world, have confirmed the correlation between cigarette smoking and lung cancer. They all concluded that smoking is responsible for 85–90 per cent of the cases of lung cancer. The risk of lung cancer increases in direct proportion to the number of cigarettes smoked per day, the number of years a person has smoked, the number of puffs per minute, the depth of inhalation, the tar content of the cigarette among other factors. The age at which a person begins smoking is also an important factor in determining the incidence of lung cancer. The risk of cancer is found to decrease progressively with time after the individual has stopped smoking. For a person who has not smoked for fifteen years, the risk of getting lung cancer is found to be only twice that of a non-smoker.

Cigarette smoking also contributes to cancers at other sites – the mouth, the larynx, the pharynx, the esophagus and the bladder. The proportion of cancer mortality in the West attributable to cigarette smoking are shown below.

> Lung 85%
> Larynx and oral cavity 50–70%
> Esophagus 50%
> Bladder and kidney 30–40%
> Pancreas 30%

It is estimated that smoking contributes to about a third of bladder cancers only; the rest come from occupational and environmental carcinogens.

Cigarette smoke contains a wide range of potent carcinogens (polycyclic aromatic hydrocarbons, N-nitrosamines), cocarcinogens and promoters (phenols), which cause cancer in the lungs, larynx, pharynx, esophagus and mouth. Cigarette smoke also contains 2-naphthalmine and 4-aminobiphenyl, which are known human bladder carcinogens. They are excreted through urine. When urine collects and remains in the bladder for some time, these carcinogens have an opportunity to exert their effects. The exact mechanism by which cigarette smoke increases the incidence of pancreatic cancer is not clear. Smoking does not contribute to cancers of the breast, colon, or prostate.

Cigarette tar contains the various carcinogens that cause smoking-related cancers. It was proved through experiments as early as in 1937, that cigarette tar causes tumours in animals.

Lung cancer is the leading cause of cancer death (accounting for a third), among both men and women in the West. In the U.K., the incidences of cancers of the larynx, mouth, pharynx and oesophagus, are low. So, the major carcinogenic effect of smoking is lung cancer, and to a lesser extent, cancers of the urinary bladder and the pancreas. The highest incidence of lung cancer among men in the world is in Scotland, 135 per 100,000. In Glasgow, lung cancer in women occurs more frequently, and is responsible for more deaths than breast cancer.

Smoking habits and patterns of cancer in India differ widely from those of the West. A far higher percentage of men in India smoke

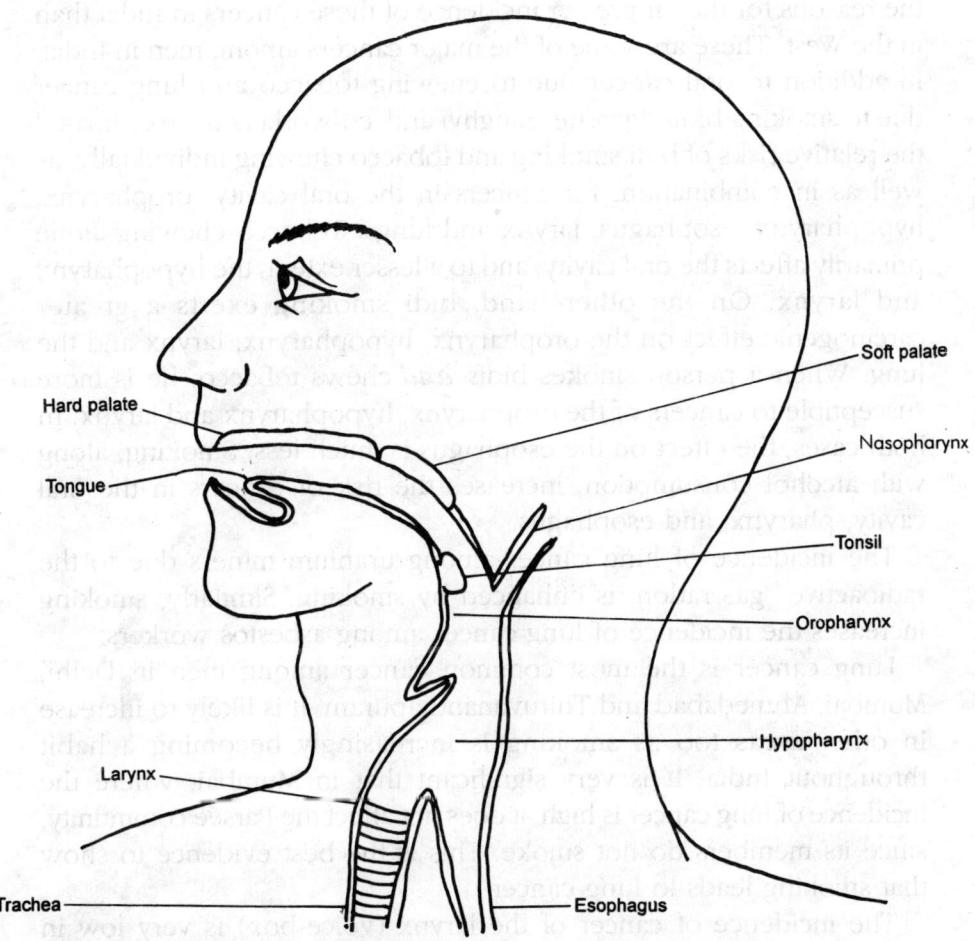

Fig. 12.1 Head and neck cancers in India

(about 50–55 per cent), compared to only 30–35 per cent in the West. Also, about 80–85 per cent of smokers smoke bidis, while only about a fifth smoke cigarettes. However this may be changing in recent years, with more and more people taking to cigarettes, due to aggressive marketing by cigarette companies. Cigarette smoking is prevalent in urban areas, among the middle and upper classes but it is now extending to rural areas.

Sanghvi and co-workers of the Tata Memorial Centre found that bidi smoking leads to cancers of the pharynx, larynx and esophagus; but its main contribution is to cancers of the oropharynx, that is, the base of the tongue (posterior third), soft palate and tonsils. Bidi smoking also leads to lung cancer. The contributions of bidi smoking to cancers of the base of the tongue, oropharynx, hypopharynx, larynx and esophagus, are greater than those of cigarette smoking. This is one of the reasons for the far greater incidence of these cancers in India than in the West. These are some of the major cancers among men in India, in addition to oral cancer due to chewing tobacco and lung cancer due to smoking bidi/cigarette. Sanghvi and co-workers have estimated the relative risks of bidi smoking and tobacco chewing individually, as well as in combination, for cancers in the oral cavity, oropharynx, hypopharynx, esophagus, larynx and lungs. Tobacco chewing alone primarily affects the oral cavity, and to a lesser extent, the hypopharynx and larynx. On the other hand, bidi smoking exerts a greater carcinogenic effect on the oropharynx, hypopharynx, larynx and the lung. When a person smokes bidis *and* chews tobacco, he is more susceptible to cancers of the oropharynx, hypopharynx and larynx. In both cases, the effect on the esophagus is much less. Smoking, along with alcohol consumption, increases the risk of cancers in the oral cavity, pharynx, and esophagus.

The incidence of lung cancer among uranium miners due to the radioactive gas radon, is enhanced by smoking. Similarly, smoking increases the incidence of lung cancer among asbestos workers.

Lung cancer is the most common cancer among men in Delhi, Mumbai, Ahmedabad and Thiruvananthapuram. It is likely to increase in other areas too as smoking is increasingly becoming a habit throughout India. It is very significant that in Mumbai, where the incidence of lung cancer is high, it does not affect the Parsee community, since its members do not smoke. This is the best evidence to show that smoking leads to lung cancer.

The incidence of cancer of the larynx (voice-box) is very low in Western countries like the U.K. and U.S.A, but is high in India, particularly in central India, where it forms 5–10 per cent of all cancers. In Gwalior and Nagpur, it is the most common kind among men. The cause of laryngeal cancer in these places is not completely known. Bidi smoking, is undoubtedly, a major contributory factor.

Cancers of the pharynx and esophagus, distinguish themselves by unusual features in their incidence. The incidence of pharyngeal cancer among men is high in the whole of eastern India. Dibrugarh in Assam has probably the highest incidence of pharyngeal cancer in the world, and accounts for nearly 30 per cent of all cancers among men there. The incidence of esophageal cancer is also high in Dibrugarh (relative frequency, 17.8 per cent). The reasons for the very high incidence of both esophageal and pharyngeal cancers in Dibrugarh have not been fully investigated so far. Smoking bidis, chewing of tobacco and the fermented areca nut, bura taamool, and drinking alcohol are possible causes. Hubli in north Karnataka also has high rates of both esophageal and pharyngeal cancers among men, each constituting about a fifth of all cancers. Esophageal cancer occurs at high rates only in isolated pockets in the world.

Cancers in the lungs, pharynx, and esophagus, are all associated with poor prognosis, and result in death, ninety per cent of the time. Hence, it is necessary to identify the important factors that cause these cancers, so that one can adopt effective preventive measures.

It is accepted that smoking causes cancer in the urinary bladder especially since cigarette smoke contains two bladder carcinogens, 2-naphthylamine and 4-aminobiphenyl. Bladder cancer is extremely common in many Western countries. In India however, high prevalence of this type of cancer occurs only among men in Jaipur and among Parsees. It is strange that it is predominant among Parsee men who do not smoke. There are, presumably, other factors, causing bladder cancer.

Smoking among women

Only 2.5 per cent of women in India, smoke since smoking among women is largely socially unacceptable. However, there are some regions, where a larger percentage of women smoke.

Reverse smoking of chuttas, a type of cigar, is widely practised by about 46 per cent of the population in the Srikakulam and Vishakhapatnam districts of Andhra Pradesh. The habit is more common among women (62 per cent). Some children also smoke chuttas. During reverse smoking, the palate heats to 58°C; where the heat acts like a cocarcinogen and accelerates the palatal changes. The changes include keratosis (diffuse whitening of the entire palatal mucosa), excrescences, that is, 1–3 mm elevated nodules; patches (well-defined, white plaques); red areas; ulceration and non-pigmented areas. Most of these changes remain for years; a small percentage regress spontaneously, but some of the red areas and patches, can become malignant. The red areas are particularly dangerous, as over half of them exhibit epithelial dysplasia and are likely to progress to cancer. Cancer of the hard palate is the primary oral cancer occurring in these regions. Cessation of smoking leads to considerable regression of the palatal changes, and primary prevention of cancer of the hard palate.

Reverse chutta smoking also affects the centre of the upper surface of the tongue, resulting in cancer. Under other conditions, oral cancer rarely occurs in the dorsum of the tongue. Cancers of the hard palate and dorsum of the tongue are almost exclusively due to reverse smoking.

Hookah smoking, practised in some parts of north India, among both men and women, is considered less harmful than bidis or cigarettes, as the smoke passes through water before reaching the smoker. Some of the toxic constituents in the smoke are retained by the water. The hookli, chilum and cigar are smoked by only a small percentage of people in India, and are becoming obsolete today.

13 Harmful Effects of Tobacco on Women and Children

Smoking kills over half a million women in the world every year. More than 75 per cent of women in Papua New Guinea smoke and about 50 per cent in Nepal smoke. About 30–35 per cent of women in Europe and North America smoke.   On the other hand, there are many countries in Africa, like Ivory Coast and Guinea, where hardly any women smoke. In India, very few women smoke. But there are some regions like Darbhanga, Goa, Simla Hills, some coastal areas of Andhra Pradesh and Orissa where smoking by women is socially acceptable, and where 25–65 per cent of women smoke.

Women in Western countries, started smoking long after men did. Well-educated, affluent women took to smoking first, more as a fashion than for any other reason. The habit was then passed on to women who were less wealthy. The affluent ladies were also the first to quit smoking, when the injurious effects of smoking became known. But the habit persists among the socially depressed women. These women who are usually less educated, unemployed, unskilled non-achievers, feel socially deprived and resort to smoking for relief.

Smoking is much more harmful to women than to men. As with men, smoking leads to chronic obstructive lung disease, ischaemic heart disease and cancer, in women too.

Causes and percentage of deaths due to smoking among women in developed countries (WHO 1985) is as follows:

Cardiovascular diseases 41%
Lung cancer 21.1%
Cancers of pharynx and larynx 2.4%
Other cancers 3.7%

COLD (Chronic bronchitis and emphysema) 18.1%

Other respiratory diseases 2.7%

Other causes 11%

Epidemiological research shows that women who use oral contraceptives *and* smoke, have a tenfold risk of heart disease. Smoking causes considerable damage to the reproductive health of women. It can produce dysmenorrhea, reduced fertility and an earlier menopause. It can also increase the risk of cancer of the cervix.

Smoking should be strictly avoided during pregnancy, as it can damage the fetus resulting in intrauterine growth retardation, low birth weight and prematurity. Smoking can cause miscarriage and stillbirth, and induce premature labour. The children born are underdeveloped, underweight, and may suffer from defective limbs.

The infant mortality is also found to be very high. If the health of the mother and the baby are already jeopardised through poverty and malnutrition, as in developing countries, the effects of smoking are likely to have an even greater impact on birth weight and perinatal mortality.

In India, about 10 per cent of women chew tobacco, and 2.5 per cent smoke, causing an estimated 17 per cent of stillbirths and 11–12 per cent of perinatal mortality. It has been estimated in 1986 that in India, nearly 457,000 deaths among infants and children under five years, could be attributed to maternal tobacco use – 124,000 stillbirths, 194,000 premature deaths, and prenatal mortality in 139,000 cases. Nicotine may be the cause of complications in pregnancy in those who smoke. Nicotine is a known vasoconstrictor and adversely affects the blood vessels in the umbilical cord. Carbon monoxide from cigarette smoke can produce anoxemia. Placental vasoconstriction can also lead to fetal anoxemia. It can deprive the fetus of other essential nutrients. Using tobacco during pregnancy seems to affect male fetuses more than female fetuses in India.

Infants with birth weight less by 100–400 g, are susceptible to infections. Premature birth and a low birth weight are often responsible for infant mortality rate in India. Since premature children suffer from inadequate physical and mental development, and frequent illness, their performance in school is only moderate. Many of them drop out of school. Those with low self-esteem, very often resort to smoking.

Passive smoking (involuntary smoking)

When a smoker does not inhale, the smoke from his cigarette (or bidi) diffuses into the surrounding atmosphere. A non-smoker who breathes this air, is said to inhale the 'sidestream'. This is known as *passive* or *involuntary smoking*. The side-stream smoke is unfiltered, containing a higher amount of tar and nicotine than the mainstream smoke inhaled by the smoker, but is diluted by air. Passive smoking has all the harmful effects of regular smoking; but at a considerably lower level. In the West where the windows are kept closed to ward off the cold, the risks of passive smoking inside the house are greater, if the inhabitants happen to be smokers. Epidemiological studies reveal that a women who does not smoke has a higher risk of lung cancer due to passive smoking than the partner of a non-smoker. This has been confirmed by innumerable studies all over the world. Hirayama, a noted Japanese epidemiologist, estimated that the passive smoker who lives with a person smoking twenty cigarettes a day, actually smokes half a cigarette per day. The risk of getting lung cancer increases progressively with the total amount of smoke taken in.

Involuntary smoking can induce cough and wheezing in an asthmatic person. Passive smoking will increase the risk of chronic respiratory disease in adults by about 25 per cent. It is very harmful to children, particularly to infants, in whom it can cause acute respiratory distress with cough, sputum, wheezing, bronchiolitis or asthma. Passive smoking will also cause both acute and chronic middle ear disease and effusions as well as sore throats. Epidemiological studies have provided ample, conclusive evidence for the causal nature of smoking for these diseases. Maternal smoking during pregnancy and after childbirth, markedly increases the chances of sudden infant death syndrome.

It is estimated that over 3000 people in the U.S.A and hundreds in Britain die of lung cancer due to passive smoking each year. To minimise passive smoking, in all the western countries, smoking in public places like schools, theaters, churches and offices is strictly forbidden. Smoking inside the houses is discouraged. In the East, Singapore and Thailand have been successful in controlling smoking. In Singapore, smoking on the roads is a punishable offence.

In India, the windows are kept open for most part of the year, and there can be free circulation of air, minimising the dangers of passive smoking. However, in flats or apartments the occupants are at risk of passive smoking. Also, while laws exist in India forbidding smoking in public places, they are not always rigorously enforced.

14 Benefits of Smoking

Recent epidemiological investigations have shown that smoking has some beneficial effects too. The benefits of smoking can be classified under four categories:

- ❑ Those which relate to women smokers only;
- ❑ Those which are due to the effects of smoking on the immune system;
- ❑ Those arising out of the action on the central nervous system;
- ❑ Those due to the effects of smoking on general metabolism.

The incidence of uterine fibroids, endometrial cancer and endometriosis is found to be considerably less among women smokers than non-smokers. Smoking is inversely related to the risk of having these gynecological disorders. The reduction in endometrial cancer is particularly pronounced in post-menopausal women but is absent in past smokers. It is well-known that these disorders are primarily due to excess estrogen. It is believed that the beneficial effects of smoking observed with regard to these diseases are due to the 'antiestrogenic' effects of smoking.

However, estrogen is necessary for maintaining the bones in the human body. Smoking, because of its antiestrogenic properties, leads to osteoporosis and hence to hip fractures and other ailments.

Chances of hypertensive disorders of pregnancy, particularly eclampsia and pre-eclampsia, can reduce by up to 30–40 per cent, with an increase in smoking. Gestational hypertension is also less common among smokers, although the effect is not so pronounced. The exact mechanism by which smoking brings about these changes is not known, though several possibilities have been suggested.

Vomiting during pregnancy is found to be less among smokers than in non-smokers though this observation is being verified. Similarly, it is not certain whether smoking women have a reduced risk of delivering infants with Down's syndrome. Several studies have found no association between cigarette smoking and breast or colon cancer.

Cigarette smoking has a profound influence on the body's immune system. It affects T-cell function, and antibody response. Hence, it reduces the incidence of some diseases, occurring due to excessive immune reaction. Three such diseases are aphthous ulcer of the oral mucosa, ulcerative colities and extrinsic allergic alveolitis.

Aphthous ulcer is characterised by tiny white spots along with ulcers occurring inside the mouth. Several studies have reported an inverse association between tobacco use and the risk of recurrent aphthous ulceration of the oral mucosa. The ulcers get worse if smoking is stopped, and get better once it is resumed. This could be due to increased oral keratinisation following tobacco use. Nicotine chewing gum is found to be equally effective.

Chronic ulcerative colitis is a painful, inflammatory condition of the colon with ulcers and bleeding. The incidence of ulcerative colitis has been repeatedly found to be much lower among current smokers than in non-smokers. The relationship between smoking and ulcerative colitis is rather complex. The risk of ulcerative colitis among ex-smokers is about the same as that of non-smokers. The symptoms of ulcerative colitis are also relieved by nicotine administration. Hence, transdermal nicotine has been administered and found to be as effective as steroids. It is found to be very helpful in treating patients with a relapse.

Extrinsic allergic alveolitis, also known as farmer's lung or bird breeder's lung, is a chronic immunologically mediated lung disorder, characterised by inflammation of the alveolus, and brought about by inhalation of allergens. The incidence of this lung disease is found to be considerably less among smokers who have lower levels of serum antibodies to the allergens responsible for this disease. Smoking probably suppresses the activity of these allergens.

While there is definite evidence that smoking has beneficial effects on aphthous ulcer, ulcerative colitis, and extrinsic allergic alveolitis, it is not certain how beneficial it is to other immunological disorders like hay fever, sarcoidosis and acne. The evidence for beneficial effects claimed is not conclusive.

Nicotine has a profound influence on the central nervous system. It resembles the most important neurotransmitter, acetylcholine, and can combine with acetylcholine receptors, either stimulating or suppressing the impulses. It liberates the neurotransmitters, noradrenaline and dopamine within the brain and can act through them.

Smoking can reduce the risk of Parkinson's disease, a neurological disorder characterised by rhythmic muscular tremors, rigid movements, odd rapid gait and drooping posture. Smokers have a relative risk of only 0.5 compared to non-smokers. Cigarette smoke or nicotine is found to ameliorate experimental Parkinsonism. Nicotine administration to patients with Parkinson's disease or several other disorders of the extrapyramidal motor system, like Tourette's syndrome, produces considerable relief.

Smoking can prevent Alzheimer's dementia too. The epidemiological evidence showing an inverse association between cigarette smoking and Alzheimer's disease is very consistent. Treatment with nicotine produces modest improvements in patients with this disease.

Smoking enhances aletrness, information processing, and memory retention in people. Administering nicotine to non-smokers is found to be equally effective in improving mental function.

The inverse relationship between body weight and smoking is well–established. The body weight of smokers has been found to be considerably lower than that of comparable non-smokers. Smoking probably increases the metabolic rate considerably and thus reduces body weight. A person who stops smoking immediately gains weight. This is one reason why smoking control programmes have not been very effective in the West, particularly among women smokers who are averse to gaining weight.

Thus, smoking has many beneficial as well as harmful effects. However, the harmful effects of smoking far outweigh its modest benefits and hence, there is urgent need for prevention of smoking. At the same time, the valuable clues provided by the study of the beneficial effects of smoking should be followed up. How far can nicotine be used for improving memory or treating Parkinson's disease. How does smoking arrest immunological disorders like ulcerative colitis? Future studies should explore if and how the beneficial effects of smoking can be secured through safer methods.

15 Psychological Effects of Smoking

The most important fact about smoking is that, people enjoy it despite being aware of its detrimental effects. This aspect should be fully appreciated by those campaigning against smoking. Reports state that animals too enjoy smoking. Monkeys which have been trained to smoke, liked inhaling cigarettes. Rats preferred to drink a dilute solution of nicotine to pure water. They were even reported to inject themselves with nicotine.

People resort to smoking for many reasons. At work, light smoking helps keep the mind aroused and alert, and improves performance. Persons, under strain, find relief in smoking. Nicotine reaches the brain within minutes of smoking, being rapidly absorbed from the lungs into the bloodstream. It causes the brain to release the neurotransmitters noradrenaline and dopamine. The limbic system in the brain contains pleasure and punishment centres. The neurotransmitters activate the pleasure centres, giving the individual a feeling of euphoria. When inhaled in large quantities, nicotine blocks the acetylcholine receptors in the punishment centre, which is responsible for unpleasant feelings like anxiety, fear, boredom, frustration, and anger. It is activated by the neurotransmitter acetylcholine. When a smoker, experiencing any such unpleasant feelings takes a deep puff, the nicotine, inhaled in large amounts, suppresses the punishment centres; the smoker is thus able to produce the desired psychological effects, by adjusting the rate and the amount of nicotine taken in.

In humans, the immediate effects of smoking or nicotine, is arousal. The electro-encephalograph (E.E.G.) shows changes typical of arousal in humans, after smoking.

In an E.E.G., alpha-waves characterised by high amplitude and low frequency, denote drowsiness; while beta-waves, with low amplitude and high frequency, indicate alertness. The varying stages of alertness range from sleep to hyperactivity, as seen below.

Stages of arousal

Sleep $\longrightarrow$ Drowsiness $\longrightarrow$ Boredom $\longrightarrow$ Relaxation $\longrightarrow$ Interest $\longrightarrow$ Alertness $\longrightarrow$ Excitement $\longrightarrow$ Hyperactivity

Smoking is found to normalise arousal, increasing it during boredom, and reducing it under stress as indicated by E.E.G. measurements. The reticular formation, a bundle of nerve fibres and cells in the brain, govern general arousal like sleep or wakefulness, or intermediary levels of arousal, while the limbic system controls a specific, goal-oriented arousal. It also determines the quality and strength of response to environmental stimuli. The neurotransmitter involved in the general arousal system is acetylcholine. As mentioned earlier, nicotine can combine with acetylcholine receptors, stimulating it when drowsy and suppressing it when excited. The limbic system is activated by the neurotransmitters, noradrenaline and dopamine. Nicotine liberates these neurotransmitters, thus activating this arousal system too.

Smoking is said to enhance learning and memory and improve productivity levels. Experiments with laboratory animals show that cigarette smoke facilitates learning and memory. Smoking activates the limbic system in the brain which is also responsible for learning and memory functions. By normalising and optimising arousal, smoking improves performance in individuals.

Tolerance: An individual's tolerance to the initial unpleasant effects of smoking increase as he continues to smoke. Many feel dizzy, nauseous, and some even vomit. After a period of time, however, the body adapts itself to smoking, by suitable methods like desensitising the vomiting centres in the brain. But the tolerance acquired is only limited, and the person might feel uneasy, if he tries to smoke a cigarette or cigar, stronger than the type he is used to. The brain always remains sensitive to smoking. An addict who resumes smoking after a day or two needs only one cigarette to drive away all the withdrawal effects and stimulate the brain.

Withdrawal syndrome: Nicotine is addictive. It initially has a pleasant, soothing effect. In course of time, it induces tolerance and dependence in the individual. Addicts, particularly those who smoke more than twenty cigarettes a day, will suffer from a withdrawal syndrome if deprived of cigarettes. Since nicotine is both a stimulant and a depressant, a person abstaining from it experiences the effects of being deprived, of both stimulatory and depressant drugs. Giving up smoking can cause difficulties in concentration, listlessness, and depression on the one hand, and anxiety, restlessness, disturbed sleep, irritability, sweating, and tremors, on the other. A heavy smoker who is deprived of cigarettes will also have an abnormally low blood pressure and a low heart rate. His E.E.G. is likely to show decreased alertness. Most abstaining smokers develop their own pattern of withdrawal syndrome which, though not life-threatening, can be severe. The most prominent withdrawal symptoms are craving and depression. Craving for cigarettes can last for months, or even years after a person quits smoking. It reaches its peak in twenty-four to forty-eight hours and then declines steadily with time. The other withdrawal symptoms are transient in nature. They reach a peak within a few days of quitting and then abate gradually, and generally disappear within a month of quitting. Most people resume smoking after quitting for a short time, primarily to avoid the withdrawal effects.

The psychological effects of smoking bidis have not been studied in great detail. The tobacco and nicotine content of a bidi, are only a fraction of that present in the cigarette. Hence, its psychological effects may be considerably fewer.

16 Smoking Habits

The factors which encourage young persons to start smoking have been extensively studied in the West. Parents, and older siblings who smoke, often induce youngsters to imitate them. Peer pressure is one of the most important reasons for adolescents taking to cigarettes. On an average, boys in the West begin smoking at twelve or thirteen. With approaching adolescence, they feel that smoking will make them appear more mature, tough and sophisticated. Smoking is found to be more prevalent among the lower socioeconomic classes, poor academic performers, and traumatised adolescents. About ninety per cent of addicts in the West are reported to have begun smoking as teenagers. The percentage of smokers among college graduates is less than that of high school graduates, which, in turn, is less than that of dropouts. Some youngsters start smoking out of sheer curiosity. Thus, social factors, particularly the environment, play a major role in inducing people to smoke.

For a beginner, the first cigarette, causes considerable irritation, nausea and unease. About thirty per cent feel sick after their first cigarette; only 20 per cent report to have enjoyed it. Persistent smoking increases tolerance, causing people to enjoy smoking without feeling nauseous. They find that smoking exhilarates them. The action of nicotine is very rapid. Once inhaled, nicotine is absorbed rapidly into the bloodstream where it moves to the brain and activates the pleasure centres. However, nicotine is metabolised very rapidly, so that within twenty to thirty minutes, the levels of nicotine in the brain and tissues fall. The smoker lights up another cigarette just to maintain high levels of nicotine in his brain and blood, and extend the feeling of euphoria. It is in this manner that most people become addicts.

People vary in their attitudes and habits when it comes to smoking. Confirmed non-smokers, will not smoke even in company. Occasional smokers, are those who are not addicts, but who smoke once in a while just to keep company. Light smokers restrict themselves to five or six cigarettes a day. Moderate smokers habitually smoke 10–25 cigarettes per day. Finally, there are the heavy smokers or chain smokers, who smoke anywhere from twenty-five to forty cigarettes a day; and are addicted to cigarettes. The moderate or heavy smoker is likely to suffer from withdrawal effects if he quits smoking. People begin smoking just for pleasure but will later smoke to avoid suffering from withdrawal symptoms. The factors responsible for a person to continue smoking are chiefly pharmacological, and are different from those responsible for inducing a person to smoke. For most drug addicts, heroin or opiates give only a short period of enjoyment, for a fortnight or a month at the beginning. The addicts then have to continue with the drugs, just to stave off the withdrawal effects. The heavy smoker is only slightly better off than the drug addict.

Smoking becomes a regular habit with many smokers. They automatically smoke a constant number of cigarettes at particular times during the day or week. In the West, most people smoke anywhere between twenty to forty cigarettes a day. In India, however, the average smoker is limited by his income, and consumes far less than twenty cigarettes a day.

There are differences in the way men and women smoke. Women take more frequent puffs of smaller volumes. The amount of nicotine obtained from a cigarette relative to the amount of tar, depends on the puffing pattern and shape. Women obtain a higher nicotine to tar ratio from each cigarette, compared to men.

Smokers alter their pattern of smoking and number of cigarettes according to their needs, and the circumstances under which they smoke. They subconsciously adjust their nicotine intake to the optimum. Smoking in company may improve the cohesiveness of social groups. When in company the smoker is relaxed, and takes in slow but deep puffs, to achieve tranquillity. When smokers have to concentrate on a demanding job and stay alert, their nicotine intake is limited to a stimulatory effect. When the addict is under stress or is agitated, he smokes many cigarettes in quick succession, taking more frequent puffs and inhaling the smoke deeply. This increases the tissue levels of nicotine which now acts as a depressant, suppressing anger, anxiety, and other such unpleasant feelings. Smoking alters (attenuates) the physiological and psychological response to stress. Thus, by subconsciously manipulating the puffs and nicotine intake, the addict is able to use smoking as a psychological tool. It stimulates him, when he is tired, helps him stay alert and aroused in a challenging task; and soothes him when he is agitated or stressed.

Unfortunately, the pleasures of smoking are short-lived, limited to the duration of the smoke. The long-term consequences of smoking, however, are serious and harmful. Habitual smoking leads to respiratory diseases, like chronic bronchitis and emphysema, cardiovascular diseases, as well as cancers at different sites, of which the most prominent is lung cancer. Addicts are reluctant to stop because while the rewards of smoking are immediate, the harmful effects of smoking are slow and appear only after many years. Besides, not all smokers suffer from the ill-effects of smoking. For example, only about 10–15 per cent of smokers get lung cancer. The fact that smoking related diseases take a long time to manifest and that not all smokers are affected, allow addicts to continue smoking, in the fond hope that they will not be affected. Thanks to the persistent, intense anti-smoking campaign in the West supported by clear, unequivocal medical evidence, about 75 per cent of smokers now admit, although half-heartedly that, cigarette smoking is very injurious to health.

Despite accepting the fact that smoking can lead to various terminal diseases, people continue smoking for various reasons. For one, they overestimate their own chances of survival, and underestimate the risks of smoking. Many of them have misconceptions about the benefits of smoking, the relative risks of smoking, and of the prognosis of smoking-related diseases. Some smokers value the psychological effects of smoking highly. They are also sceptical of anti-smoking campaings, and the information on the effects of smoking on one's health. But there are smokers who genuinely believe that smoking is very bad for health. Many have tried to quit smoking but only a few succeed, because of the addictive nature of nicotine. Only one of four smokers trying to quit, succeeds in doing so.

In course of time, addicts begin experiencing some of the unpleasant effects of smoking. These include coughs, dyspnea, sore throats, respiratory infections, symptoms of peptic ulcer, oesophagitis, angina, dental and gum diseases, and so on. It is then that they realise, that they are not immune to the long-term effects of smoking, and start thinking about quitting. When some of these symptoms become severe they feel the need to quit smoking. Many may attempt to quit but very few succeed. The craving for cigarettes, and the withdrawal symptoms following abstinence, compel them to go back to smoking unless they have good self-control.

Several strategies have been devised to help addicts quit smoking. These include *counselling* by the family physician, *treatment* of withdrawal effects with drugs, particularly nicotine chewing gum *behaviour therapy hypnosis*, and so on. A number of *smoking clinics* have now opened in the West, to help people quit smoking. Counselling by physicians helps tremendously. It is enough if the physician spends three to five minutes with the smoker, patiently explaining to him the long-term benefits of quitting – better health and greater longevity. The quitting rate is found to be double when the physician takes a personal interest in helping an addict quit smoking. The family physician's role includes: boosting the smoker's resolve to quit, helping the smoker overcome his withdrawal syndrome by prescribing suitable drugs, particularly nicotine chewing gum, encouraging the smoker to try again, if he relapses. Counselling by the family physician is also found to be cost-effective.

Nicotine chewing gum

The main incentive in smoking is the consumption of nicotine, and the major impediment for quitting is the withdrawal syndrome, brought about by nicotine deficiency. Hence, it would be logical to attempt nicotine administration as an alternative to smoking. Initially, nicotine was administered orally in the form of nicotine tartarate tablets and found to be completely ineffective, since the blood level was too low. Nicotine chewing gum has been found to be far more satisfactory and is widely used now.

Nicotine chewing gum is a resin containing 2 mg of nicotine and a bicarbonate buffer. A spicy flavour masks the taste and irritating sensation of nicotine. The bicarbonate buffer provides an alkaline medium, allowing for greater absorption of nicotine. The gum should be chewed very slowly, for over twenty to thirty minutes so that the nicotine is gradually released and completely absorbed through the buccal mucosa into the bloodstream. The blood level of nicotine attained is about a third to half of that produced by smoking cigarettes. The withdrawal symptoms are considerably reduced, though not completely eliminated. Nicotine gum is particularly useful for those smokers who had withdrawal symptoms earlier, those who smoke within thirty minutes of waking up and those who smoke even when they are sick. There are several reports that nicotine gum helps a person abstain from cigarettes.

Nicotine gum however, has some minor side-effects related to chewing and to the influence of nicotine on the gastrointestinal system. It can cause irritation in the mouth, sore jaws, sore throat, heartburn, dyspepsia and hiccups. Dental appliances such as bridges and caps can occasionally loosen or deteriorate. A few patients also experience palpitations.

Nicotine gum should be used correctly to derive maximum benefit and minimise potential unpleasant side-effects. Because it is meant only to relieve withdrawal effects, the gum has to be regularly used, only after the patient has stopped smoking. It is imperative that the patient chews the gum slowly, because vigorous chewing will result in nicotine being released too quickly, and this irritates the mouth. Excess nicotine is swallowed, as its absorption through the buccal mucosa is slow. As it passes through the gastrointestinal tract, it causes hiccups, heartburn, belching, nausea, and dyspepsia. It is primarily metabolised and inactivated in the liver, and very little reaches the bloodstream to produce any psychological effect. A smoker trying to quit, should use this gum for at least three months and chew it as soon as she feels a desire to smoke. Many people stop using nicotine gum as soon as they feel confident that they can do without it. A few become addicted to it and use it for as long as one year.

The use of nicotine gum is contraindicated during pregnancy and in cases of recent myocardial infarction, and life-threatening arrhythmias. Nicotine gum may aggravate coronary disease, peptic ulcers, esophagitis and peripheral vascular diseases. Hence, care should be exercised in prescribing it to the patient.

Other drugs: Many other drugs have been tried to relieve withdrawal effects but have not been of much use. These include lobeline and tranquillisers like diazepam. The opiate antagonist naloxane is very effective but the effect does not last long. Chloridine, an anti-hypertensive drug and an alpha-adrenergic antagonist relieves a number of acute withdrawal effects in heavy smokers. A dosage of 0.15–0.30 mg of chloridine per day has been found to benefit heavy smokers receiving behavioural therapy. However, its long-term effects are not known.

Aversion therapy: Two forms of aversion therapy are being practised, both of which are unpleasant. In one, the addict receives a mild electric shock, whenever he tries to light or pick up a cigarette, or even when he expresses a desire to smoke. In the other, the addict is made to smoke rapidly, about one puff in six seconds, a rate much faster than what she is accustomed to. Both these forms of treatment induce a strong dislike for smoking in the addict. The second method is said to have a success rate of 60 per cent.

Hypnosis: Hypnosis is one of the most popular methods to stop addicts from smoking. It is also found to be very effective. This method will be successful only under certain conditions:

❑   The patient should be strongly motivated to give up smoking.

- ❑ The therapy should be individualised, taking into consideration the particular patient's mental makeup.
- ❑ The treatment should involve a number of sessions and regular follow-up.

Acupuncture: Acupuncture, as a method for quitting smoking, has not been studied fully. It has been claimed that acupuncture produces an immediate, strong dislike for the taste and smell of tobacco. This claim, however, needs confirmation and thorough investigation.

Smoking clinics: A number of smoking clinics exist in the West to help addicts give up smoking. Besides educating them about the evils of smoking and techniques to quit the habit, they also offer a wide range of treatment like counselling (psychiatric treatment), hypnosis, group therapy and 'programmed smoking'. They advise addicts on using nicotine chewing gum correctly. Smokers derive some benefit from these clinics but the success rates is only a moderate (about 12 to 28 per cent).

Relapse: Most of the cessation methods practised, initially cause a substantial decrease or even an outright elimination of smoking. But this success is very short-lived. *Relapse is the most important problem with smoking.* There is a steep decline in the number of non-smokers, so that by the end of three months, only about 35 per cent remain non-smokers, and at the end of six months, only 25 per cent. After this period, the number of non-smokers reverting to smoking is less, so that at the end of one year, about 20 per cent remain non-smokers. Generally, they continue as non-smokers so that the true success rate is about 20 per cent.

Men are more successful in quitting smoking than women. This may be because men and women smoke for different reasons. While most men smoke for relaxation, and as a pastime, women smoke generally start smoking to soothe themselves, to attenuate their anger or anxiety and decrease their stress. Smoking that is started in order to provide relief from stress, is more difficult to quit.

Surveys conducted also reveal that people who have not had much exposure to cigarette smoke, find it easier to quit. These include light smokers, those who have been smoking only for a short time, and those who do not inhale smoke from a cigarette. Extroverts and people with better education, are also found to be more successful in quitting.

Will power and self-control are absolutely necessary for a person to quit smoking. A majority of those who have successfully quit smoking, have accomplished it through self-control alone.

17 The Rise and Fall of the Cigarette in the West

The rise of the cigarette

The cigarette originated in Central or North America during the nineteenth century. There is no record of who invented it, or whether it evolved in the course of time. The cigarette is now smoked by all races in all the countries of the world. Europeans were introduced to the cigarette during the Crimean War, (1856–1858). The automatic cigarette making machine which was invented in 1853, made cigarettes easily available at very low cost. Very soon, it replaced the cigar and the pipe as the most convenient form of smoking. At about the same time, many governments enacted legislation prohibiting tobacco chewers from spitting in public areas. Tobacco addicts took to cigarette smoking instead. World War I (1914–1918) provided a very great impetus for the spread of cigarettes. The soldiers took to smoking to relax, and to break the monotony while waiting at the battlefront. Smoking among women was socially unacceptable until World War I, when women's rights activists began smoking in an attempt to campaign for equality with men. By 1950, smoking became popular among both men and women in the West. Cigarette smoking became widespread. People smoked for various reasons – for relaxation, to stimulate themselves and remain alert at work, to tone down their anger and to soothe themselves when depressed.

Discovery of the harmful effects of cigarettes

By the close of the nineteeth century, people became dimly aware that smoking could cause respiratory disorders. In 1938, Professor Pearl of the Johns Hopkins Institute provided convincing statistical evidence that cigarettes could reduce a person's longevity.

The announcement came as an eye-opener, showing people that cigarette smoking may not be as beneficial as they thought it was. This had two important consequences. First, a thorough analysis of the chemical constituents of cigarette smoke and their biological effects was undertaken. This revealed that cigarette smoke contains numerous harmful chemicals – carbon monoxide, which interferes with oxygen transport and contributes to ischemic heart disease; hydrogen cyanide, a potent cilia poison leading to bronchitis; nicotine, which increases pulse rate and heart rate, and contributes to coronary heart disease; a wide range of carcinogens, cocarcinogens, and tumour promoters including the volatile N-nitrosamines, non-volatile tobacco-specific nitrosamines, the potent polycyclic aromatic hydrocarbons, and small amounts of the radioactive polonium-210. Simultaneously, large-scale epidemiological investigations on the health effects of smoking were carried out, involving a number of case-control and prospective studies. The results revealed that smoking can cause cancers in various parts of the body such as the lungs, mouth, larynx, pharynx, esophagus, pancreas, kidney and bladder. Smoking can also give rise to some non-fatal but very distressing diseases like peripheral vascular disease, cataract, hip fracture and periodontal disease. Smoking during pregnancy can harm the fetus. The fetus is also succeptible to spontaneous abortion, ectopic pregnancy, limb reduction defects, low birth weight, stillbirth and neonatal death. The first report on Smoking and Health by the Royal College of Physicians, London in 1962 and the U.S. Surgeon-General's Report in 1964, clearly brought out these harmful effects of smoking. They were confirmed in subsequent reports of the U.S. Surgeon-General. Passive smoking, particularly in poorly ventilated rooms and confined spaces, was also found to be very injurious. These reports concluded that a fifth of all deaths in these countries were due to smoking alone, an enormous loss of life, which is strictly preventable.

Restrictions on cigarette smoking

These revelations on the deleterious effects of smoking had a powerful impact on the public, the media, the government as well as the cigarette manufacturing companies. As it could not be banned outright in any free society, governments took a wide range of measures to curb smoking. Excise duty on tobacco and cigarettes was raised. It was found that a tax rise of 10 per cent resulted in only a one per cent decrease in the number of smokers. Smoking in public places such as theatres, cinemas, churches and offices was banned. Open advertising and promotion of cigarettes and other tobacco products were forbidden on television and restricted in other media. The government also made it compulsory to mention on every cigaratte packet, the public health warning `cigarette smoking is very injuries to health'. Smokers were helped in their attempts to quit smoking by increasing the number of Smoking withdrawal clinics, and subsidising anti-smoking aids and anti-smoking campaigns.

Filter cigarettes

Cigarette manufacturing companies responded to the increased awareness of smoking among the public, by introducing well-ventilated, filter cigarettes covered with perforated paper. This helped to reduce the levels of tar, carbon monoxide, and other toxic constituents of cigarette smoke. By using suitable blends of tobacco and changing their manufacturing patterns, the tar and nicotine contents of cigarettes have been progressively reduced to 10–15 mg tar and 1.3–1.5 mg nicotine per cigarette. This is found to be the minimum acceptable level of nicotine, for smokers. Low-tar, low-nicotine cigarettes yielding just 10 mg tar and 1 mg nicotine, are also available. Some governments also stipulate that the tar and nicotine yields of cigarettes should also be displayed on the cigarette packet. Smoking low-tar, low-nicotine filter cigarettes substantially reduces the incidence of lung cancer.

Compensatory smoking

When low-tar, low-nicotine filter cigarettes were introduced, the smoker adopted various strategies to compensate for the lower nicotine yield of cigarettes, and to get the usual amount of nicotines she was accustomed to. She increased the number of cigarettes smoked, and the number of puffs taken from each cigarette. In such cigarettes, a larger volume of smoke is taken from each puff, and inhaled more deeply. The cigarettes are also smoked to a shorter butt-length. By adopting all these measures, the smoker was able to compensate for nearly two-thirds of the nicotine decrease due to low-tar, low-nicotine cigarettes. A 35 per cent reduction in nicotine resulted in an 18 per cent increase in the number of cigarettes smoked. Despite this, however, low-tar, low-nicotine cigarettes helped in substantially lowering the incidence of lung cancer. *But the risk still remains; there is no such thing as a safe cigarette.*

Decline in smoking among men and women

Following the reports in the early 1960s of the Royal College of Physicians, U.K. and the Surgeon-General, U.S.A, the media in these countries began carrying out intense anti-smoking campaigns very effectively. The proportion of men smoking started declining first. The percentage of Americans smoking decreased from 64 per cent in the 1950s to about 31 per cent in 1990. The decrease in the consumption of cigarettes among men in the U.K. fell from about 98 billion in 1986 to 91 billion pieces in 1992/93. Because of a lag period of twenty to thirty years between smoking and the onset of lung cancer, the decline in the incidence of lung cancer among men came much later. The incidence of lung cancer among men steadily increased for a number of years, from 20 per 100,000 persons in 1950 to 70 per 100,000 in 1975, stabilised to 75 per 100,000 in 1985, then began decreasing.

Women started smoking later; and the proportion of women smoking steadily increased, even after men had started quitting. The decline in smoking among women occurred only recently. The incidence of lung cancer among women in U.S.A. has been steadily increasing from 5 per 100,000 persons to 25 per 100,000 from 1960 to 1985; and has started stabilising only recently. The second half of the twentieth century thus witnessed a steady decrease in consumption of cigarettes in Western Europe and the United States.

According to the latest reports from the U.S.A. (March 1999), smoking is no longer a socially acceptable practice. Cigarette smoking is progressively declining and may soon become completely extinct in the U.S.A.. In Britain, the medical profession gave up smoking first. Medical students no longer smoke. Some Scandinavian countries are planning to have a completely smoke-free generation.

Dumping of cigarettes in third world countries

The manufacture and marketing of cigarettes is controlled by about seven multinational companies, based mainly in the U.S.A. and U.K. On finding that their markets have shrunk in the developed countries, these companies have started dumping cigarettes on the third world countries in Asia, Africa and South America. Through aggressive marketing tactics, they have already established themselves in most of the countries and started making huge profits. Though smoking inside the U.S.A. is actively discouraged, the production of tobacco in the U.S.A. has actually increased from about 600,000 to 700,000 tons per year between 1985 and 1994. So also the manufacture of cigarettes. Cigarette smoking has been on the rise in third world countries even as it is decreasing in Western Europe and the United States. The opening decades of the twenty-first century will witness a very rapid increase in lung cancer, almost to epidemic proportions, in the developing countries. Hopefully, this may be followed by a decline in the rate of cigarette consumption and lung cancer.

18 Global Efforts at Tobacco Control

Medical and economic impact of tobacco use

It is now accepted all over the world that smoking is the single major avoidable cause of disease, debility and death. About three million people in the world die of tobacco-related diseases every year, out of the eleven million people suffering from them.

Using tobacco products also creates economic losses, for the consumer, government and society. The diagnosis and treatment of these diseases, particularly cancer, are very expensive, and pose a huge economic burden on the patients and their families, and if subsidised, on the government and the society. Imported cigarettes will bring about a huge drain on foreign exchange.

Tobacco is sometimes cultivated on land which could be better used to grow food grains. Curing of tobacco involves using large amounts of wood, which in turn, leads to large-scale deforestation. Using cigarettes carelessly can cause fires, and cigarette smoke pollutes the atmosphere.

COMPOSITE PROGRAMME FOR TOBACCO CONTROL

In the early 1960s, the discovery of a close link between cigarette smoking, lung cancer and various other diseases, brought about public concern. The media and the governments, were forced to adopt several measures to control cigarette smoking, and restrict tobacco use. The W.H.O. evolved a comprehensive, composite, tobacco control programme whose major objectives were:

- ❑ To prevent persons from starting to smoke;
- ❑ To help addicts to quit smoking;

❏ To reduce the toxic constituents in cigarette smoke, and hence minimise the damage to smokers who are unable to quit;
❏ To protect non-smokers from environmental smoke.

This composite programme has several arms; these are listed below.

MASS HEALTH EDUCATION

This attempts to raise public awareness about the adverse effects of smoking, chewing tobacco and dipping snuff, by using the mass media. The ultimate goal of this method is to create a well-informed society, where non-smoking would be the norm. The publication of the 1962 and 1971 reports of the Royal College of Physicians of London started a reversal in the trend and greatly contributed to the 30 per cent decline in male smoking in the U.K. (1962–1980). Similarly, the periodical publication of the U.S. Surgeon-General's Reports from 1964 onwards is a major contributory factor in the decline of smoking prevalence in the U.S.A. Large-scale health education through the media helps prevent non-smokers from taking to cigarettes. In a habitual smoker, it also substantially increases the motivation to quit. Equally important, it facilitates necessary legislation such as increasing tax rates, to control smoking.

Educating the public through the mass media on the adverse effects of smoking, is a prime requisite for any tobacco control programme.

BAN ON ALL FORMS OF TOBACCO ADVERTISEMENTS AND PROMOTION

Most children and teenagers are lured by cigarette advertisements, which depict the smoker possessing mature, tough qualities, which they themselves would like to emulate. The tobacco industry is extremely resourceful in designing advertisements to attract specific groups. For example, it had brought out *slim cigarettes* to encourage smoking among young girls. Once a person becomes a smoker, he or she finds it extremely difficult to quit. Even with all the cessation techniques available now, only about 35 per cent of smokers are able to quit smoking. The saying once a smoker, always a smoker generally holds true. Hence, we need to prevent the urge to smoke in the first place. Banning all forms of tobacco advertisement will be of great help.

Multinational tobacco companies who have money and influence, also engage themselves in numerous promotional activities, sponsoring games and entertainment programmes so on. This indirectly serves in promoting their product. It also creates a circle of people who become dependent on the tobacco industry for funds.

Realising the serious consequences of tobacco advertising and promoting, twenty-seven countries have banned outright all forms of tobacco advertisements and promotional activities. Eighty-four countries have imposed severe restrictions on tobacco advertising. All these countries have prohibited the sale of cigarettes to minors.

Health warnings

Most countries stipulate that every cigarette packet should carry the health warning 'cigarette smoking is injurious to health'. This warning is carried even in those countries where cigarette advertising has not been banned. In practice, however, this single line advertisement is barely noticeable. This warning also has no effect on the addict, who becomes used to seeing it. However, it may influence a young potential smoker. It may also counteract promotional advertisements.

There have been many suggestions to make this health warning large, and hence effective. A few advanced countries stipulate that the tar and nicotine yields of the cigarettes should also be printed on the packets.

Strategies for cessation of smoking

A variety of cessation techniques can be employed to help smokers quit, depending on their motivation and degree of addiction.

Smokers attempt to quit only after making a conscious decision to do so. However it has been observed that less than five per cent of smokers succeed in abstaining from cigarettes at the end of a year. It is thus necessary to help smokers quit if the success rate is to be appreciable.

Brief counselling sessions for three to five minutes by the family physician is found to help light smokers. Apart from counselling them on the beneficial health effects of quitting, the physician may also provide leaflets on the hazards of smoking. The success rate achieved is limited, only 5–12 per cent. Greater success can be achieved through longer sessions but this may not be cost-effective. The distribution of free nicotine gum or a nicotine patch substantially increases the quit rate, and prevents quitters from relapsing.

Counselling alone is not enough for moderate smokers to quit. Such smokers use fifteen or more cigarettes a day, and start smoking within thirty minutes of waking up. More than half of them will experience withdrawal symptoms, when they try to quit and need nicotine replacement either in the form of nicotine gum or transdermal nicotine patches which are now easily available and can be used during the day, or for 24 hours. With only a few side-effects, they are best for brief use. The physician should guide the smoker about using nicotine chewing gum properly. The gum should be chewed very slowly for twenty to thirty minutes, so that the nicotine is gradually released, and absorbed through the buccal mucosa into the bloodstream. Nicotine nasal sprays cause irritation in the nose, and have poor compliance. They are useful for highly addicted, heavy smokers. Nicotine replacement therapy has been found to help moderate to heavy smokers and prevent them from having a relapse. Some moderate smokers, treated with nicotine patches, can quit smoking within a week. The nicotine patch treatment is very cost-effective for these patients.

Highly motivated, but addicted heavy smokers, need intensive therapy in specialised clinics to help them quit smoking. The treatment is very expensive, involving repeated counselling in many sessions, nicotine replacements in various forms, and so on. Group therapies are arranged to save physician's time, and cost to the smoker. Patients attending specialised clinics within a particular geographical area, are grouped together or paired within the group, and made to declare their commitment to abstinence.They are then offered treatment through various cessation techniques. They are often made to check upon each other to ensure that all addicts maintain abstinence. Smoking by any defaulter can be easily checked through two biochemical parameters: by measuring the nicotine metabolite cotinine levels in the saliva (this test is applicable only for those not receiving any nicotine replacement like nicotine gum) and by measuring carbon monoxide in the expired air. Expired carbon monoxide is found to be a useful indicator of smoking in 90 per cent of cases. Portable carbon monoxide meters are now available. Intensive treatment in 'specialist smokers clinics' resulted in 35 per cent of abstainers at the end of one year; and 22 per cent at 5 years, compared to 9 per cent and 5 per cent respectively in the non-intervention group.

FISCAL POLICY

One of the most effective ways of reducing smoking is to raise the taxes on tobacco and tobacco products. For every 10 per cent increase in tax in U.S.A., there is a four per cent decrease of adult smokers and a 14 per cent decrease of teenage smokers. Governments raise tax on tobacco and tobacco products for three reasons: to raise their total revenue, to compensate for medical and health care expenses arising out of tobacco-related diseases and to curb smoking (sumptuary tax).

In Western countries, smoking is closely linked to the socioeconomic group. Over half of the people in the lowest socioeconomic group (unskilled manual workers, and their spouses, smoke). They also suffer most from tobacco-related diseases such as chronic obstructive lung disease, ischemic heart disease and lung cancer. The price rise in tobacco and cigarette has its maximum impact on this group producing a sharp decline in the number of cigarettes smoked. Smoking in the upper socioeconomic groups (professional workers, managers, and their spouses), is not a major problem and any price rise in cigarettes or tobacco has no effect on their smoking behaviour. Smoking is moderate in the middle socioeconomic groups (clerical workers, skilled and semi-skilled manual workers), and they also respond moderately to price rise in cigarettes and tobacco. It has been reported that the government revenue increases even though the overall consumption of cigarettes falls. The increase in tobacco tax is borne more by the wealthier smokers than the poorer ones sincethey can afford to smoke at the same level as before.

The prevalence of smoking is highest among the poor, who spend a disproportionate share of their incomes on smoking. Any reduction in their smoking due to a price rise in cigarettes, will benefit their own and their families' health. However, addicts who continue with their smoking at the same level as before will be spending a lot more on cigarettes than earlier. Thus, price rise in cigarettes can damage many poor families. Governments will have to carefully monitor its taxation on tobacco and tobacco products, out of consideration for socially disadvantaged groups. A method of progressive taxation on tobacco and tobacco products is one of the key elements in the Comprehensive Tobacco Control Programme administered by the World Health Organization. An efficient fiscal policy on tobacco, coupled with sound mass health education achieves the maximum results. As the majority of people are non-smokers, and as the whole society is fully aware of the harmful effects of smoking, tax on cigarettes for health reasons, is a popular tax, enthusiastically accepted by most sections of society in the West.

There are some countries in Europe, where hand-rolled cigarettes are used. They include the Netherlands (49 per cent of all consumption); Denmark (27 per cent), Belgium (21 per cent), Germany (10 per cent), France   (5 per cent) and the U.K. (4 per cent). These cigarettes are taxed less but have a higher tar yield. All these will adversely affect tobacco control in these countries.

PRODUCT MODIFICATION

The established correlation between cigarettes and a number of serious diseases, as well as the knowledge that cigarettes are addictive brought about various programmes to control and prevent smoking. From early 1970s progressive product modification with less and less toxic yields became an integral part of all comprehensive tobacco control programmes.

Tobacco companies responded by introducing filter cigarettes, with substantially reduced tar and nicotine yields. Since the reduction in both these substances were gradual and spread over years, they did not evoke any consumer resistance. By 1993, the tar yield of cigarettes in the U.K. had been reduced to 15 mg/cigarette. It was agreed that, by 1997, the upper limit for tar would be 12 mg/cigarette, and for nicotine 1 mg/cigarette. This will be followed by all countries of the European Union (EU).

Deaths due to lung cancer and chronic obstructive lung disease have been substantially reduced by product modification. The effect on ischemic heart disease has not yet been clearly established.

BAN ON SMOKING IN PUBLIC PLACES

The majority of people are non-smokers and should be protected from environmental tobacco smoke. Passive smoking can also cause respiratory distress, lung cancer and other diseases. Hence, many countries have banned smoking in public places like schools, churches, and theaters. Smoking is also either completely banned or largely restricted in most of the larger companies and other workplaces in the U.K.

CONTROL OF TOBACCO HABITS IN DEVELOPED COUNTRIES

Among the Western countries, the U.K. and the U.S.A. have made remarkable progress in controlling smoking among both men and women, by adopting the comprehensive tobacco control programme initiated by the W.H.O. Smoking among men declined steadily from about 60 per cent in 1960 to about 28–30 per cent in 1992 in the U.K. Smoking among women rose steadily from about 38 per cent in 1950 to 45 per cent in 1966–70, and has steadily decreased since then to 28 per cent in 1992. Though a steady decline in adult smoking has been achieved in the U.K., the rates of smoking among teenagers are still high. About one in four teenagers become addicts by the time they reach sixteen. The U.K. hopes to reduce the rate of adult smoking from about 30 per cent in 1990 to 20 per cent by 2000, reduce underage smoking from 8 per cent to less than 6 per cent of 11–15 year-olds, and smoking during pregnancy, by about a third.

Scotland has one of the highest incidences of smoking and lung cancer, among both men and women. Anti-smoking measures, including counselling through telephones, are now being pursued vigorously.

In the U.S.A., while smoking has been on the decline, there has been a revival of the use of smokeless tobacco. From the 1970s, teenagers and young adults have been increasingly chewing tobacco and dipping snuff. These practices are more common among boys than girls. Smokeless tobacco causes leukoplakia, and oral and pharyngeal cancers. The five-year survival for oral and pharyngeal cancers is about 50 per cent in the U.S.A. As such, the morbidity and mortality associated with smokeless tobacco is considerably less than that in smoking. Smokeless tobacco is still popular among native Americans. About a third of them use smokeless tobacco, and are consequent victims to oral lesions.

Tobacco control programmes are being pursued very seriously in some Scandinavian countries like Norway and Sweden. These countries use *rotating health warning* on packets of cigarettes and other tobacco products. In this system of rotating warnings, several different messages are in use at any one moment, appearing at random on all packages and on advertisements. Norway and Sweden each use sixteen warnings and periodically replaced them with a new set to ensure that the messages remain effective.

Tobacco control programmes in many other European countries are not as advanced as those in the U.K. or U.S.A. While lung cancer has been decreasing in the U.K. Since 1988, it has more than doubled in Yugoslavia, Poland, and Hungary. Lung cancer mortality has increased by 55 per cent in the former U.S.S.R. between 1970 and 1980. In some of the European countries, women have begun smoking only recently. In many countries in Eastern Europe, which have recently become free from communist rule, state monopoly trading in tobacco has ended. Multinational tobacco companies have entered these new markets, after buying many local companies there. A steady rise in smoking and lung cancer in these countries can be expected in the coming decades.

CONTROL OF TOBACCO HABITS IN DEVELOPING COUNTRIES

With a population of over one billion, China has the highest number of cigarette smokers in the world. More than half of the men, but only 6 per cent of women, smoke. The most popular form of smoking is cigarettes. So China has been the biggest target of all multinational cigarette companies for decades. Till recently, there was monopolistic trading by Chinese National Tobacco Corporation, but now the Chinese market has been thrown open and multinational companies are reported to have already started advertising there, though China has passed a comprehensive tobacco control legislation. It would be interesting to see how this country fares in the next few decades.

There are wide differences among developing countries with regard to tobacco control. Some countries like Thailand, Singapore, Sudan and Botswana, have stringent tobacco control programmes, which are strictly implemented. Even multinational tobacco companies are punished, if they violate these regulations. However, there are also many countries, particularly in Africa, where very few men and women smoke. These countries do not even have a national survey of tobacco habits or any programme for tobacco control. They are not fully aware of all the harmful effects of smoking, or of the various strategies adopted by multinational cigarette companies to spread this habit.

Tobacco companies spend billions of dollars to advertise their products, and counteract the growing public awareness of smoking. Advertising and other promotional techniques used in developing countries are reported to be different from those used in developed countries with strict tobacco control programmes. Tobacco companies are accused of following double standards.

The risk of tobacco-related diseases in developing countries is rising due to increased consumption of manufactured cigarettes. Between 1970 and 1980, cigarette consumption increased by 62.5 per cent in Pakistan, by 40 per cent in India; by 32 per cent in Kenya but by only 4 per cent in the U.S.A. In the U.K., cigarette consumption was actually decreasing. Asia now accounts for more than half of world's consumption of cigarettes. Lung cancer is one of the three commonest forms of cancer in India, Malaysia, and Pakistan, and is common among both blacks and whites in Zimbabwe. Tobacco-related diseases will appear in developing countries in a very big way, even before communicable diseases and malnutrition have been controlled. This is in sharp contrast to the West, where communicable diseases and malnutrition are no longer present. Thus, the health problems of the third world countries will be far more severe, unless remedial measures are taken immediately.

There are many international organisations, which are concerned about the health hazards of tobacco habits and the impact of tobacco control programmes. Some of them are the World Health Organization (W.H.O.); the International Union against Cancer (U.I.C.C.); International Union against Tuberculosis and Lung Diseases; International Agency on Tobacco and Health; Action on Smoking and

Health; International Organisation of Consumer Unions; International Network of Women Against Tobacco, and Asia Pacific Association for the Control of Tobacco (A.S.P.A.C.T.). There are many others, all of which work towards safeguarding the health and well-being of humanity.

19 Tobacco Control in India

The developed and developing countries who have realised the harmful effects of smoking and chewing tobacco, are striving hard to control the rates of tobacco consumption. Though none of them will achieve the WHO goal of *'Health for all by 2000 A.D.'*, they would have gone a long way towards that end. In India however, there have been very few measures taken to control tobacco consumption. Numerous factors, economic, social, and others, make it difficult to implement tobacco control programmes in India.

Firstly, the cultivation and manufacture of tobacco products play an important role in the Indian economy. India is the third largest producer of tobacco in the world, after China and U.S.A. It produces 587 million kg of tobacco annually, in 391,000 hectares of land. The tobacco industry in India is also very well-established producing a variety of tobacco products like bidis, cigarettes, hookah paste, zarda, cigars, cheroots and chuttas. Raw FCV (flue-cured Virginia) tobacco is exported to the U.K., Russia, Japan, Italy and Iraq. Manufactured tobacco is exported to countries in the Middle East. All these provide the government of India with an appreciable excise duty (Rs. 3,445.82 crores during 1994–95) and foreign exchange (Rs. 421 crores during 1995–96). The Indian government is thus reluctant to take steps that would cut down on these revenues.

Tobacco is a highly remunerative crop, and gives good returns. However, as most farmers sell their products during harvest season for want of the storage facilities, the crop is sold at extremely low prices. The major share of the profits go to merchants and middlemen. Since other crops are not as remunerative as tobacco, or as rugged and pest-resistant, tobacco cultivators are reluctant to switch to other crops. People employed in the manufacture, packing, distribution, export, and sale of tobacco products, reap high profits, and are hence averse to tobacco control.

Secondly, the Indian tobacco industry employs five to six million persons. About 1.2 million people are engaged in the cultivation, processing, and curing of tobacco, and another 3 million (including illiterate women in rural areas) in the manufacture of bidi. Thousands of tribals are employed in the collection of bidi leaves. The cigarette industry alone provides employment to 25,000 people, while 500,000 people are engaged in the marketing and export of tobacco and tobacco products. Thus, any attempt at tobacco control will affect millions of people, including socially disadvantaged groups like women and tribals. Any elected government, will think twice before creating such social upheaval. Tobacco control in India must necessarily be gradual.

Society's attitude towards smoking is an important factor determining the success of any anti-smoking campaign. Smoking is now an accepted practice in India, unlike sixty years ago, when it was a social taboo. A majority of people, including many educated people, are not aware of all the serious ill-effects of smoking. Cinema also often depicts smoking. This is in sharp contrast to the U.S.A, where public figures refuse to appear with a cigarette in hand. The Indian public has to be educated about the highly deleterious effects of smoking, the variety of diseases it can cause, and the fatal nature of many of them if we are to implement any tobacco control programme.

The government of India exerts some control over the manufacture, promotion, and sale of tobacco products (primarily cigarettes) but not very effectively. It has enacted the Cigarette Act, 1975, which stipulates that all cartons and packets of cigarettes, and advertisements should carry the statutory warning, 'Cigarette smoking is injurious to health'. Cigarettes carry higher tax but any increase in the rate of tax will have only a marginal effect, as only the affluent smoke cigarettes. Others may cut down slightly on the number of cigarettes they smoke. Cigarette packets and advertisements carry the statutory warning, but as the cigarette companies themselves are fully aware, this warning has practically no effect on smokers. All cigarettes sold in India including the so-called filter cigarettes, are reported to have high yield of tar and nicotine. An average Indian cigarette contains 19–28 mg tar and up to 1.8 mg nicotine as compared to tar and nicotine yields of 12 mg and 1 mg per cigarette in the U.K. It is unfortunate that there is no legislation or any move to control these levels.

There are absolutely no restrictions on cigarette advertising in India, except in state-controlled radio and T.V. channels. Most small shops in Tamil Nadu, for example, carry large signboards advertising cigarette brands. After the economic reforms of the early nineties, foreign brands have also started making their appearance in the Indian market.

As bidis are a product of a cottage industry, its employees enjoy several concessions from the Indian government. While cigarettes are subject to progressive rises in tax, the excise duty on bidis is still comparatively low. Packets of bidis and tobacco do not carry any health warning, despite the fact that bidis contain higher levels of tar and nicotine than cigarettes. Epidemiological studies reveal that cancers of the larynx and pharynx are more common in India than in the West, because of the high rates of bidi consumption. There is practically no quality control on the tobacco used for chewing and making bidis. Millions of dollars are spent on promoting cigarettes, which are subject to some government restriction. On the other hand, there is very little promotion for bidis or chewing tobacco. Bidis act as cheap alternatives for cigarettes and in a way, stem the rapid spread of cigarettes, backed by multinational cigarette companies. Bidi smoking in India is confined to people of the lower middle-class and the poor.

The use of tobacco preparations as dentifrices is another feature unique to India. Many popular brands of toothpastes in Bombay and Goa contain tobacco. Their long-term use will certainly lead to oral lesions, including cancer.

Smoking in public places like schools, hospitals, cinemas, religious places, buses and airlines should be strictly prohibited. Recently, the government has banned the sale of cigarettes in railway stations. Smoking inside government offices and institutions has also been banned.

While the general public are only now waking up to the consequences of using tobacco, the doctors in India have been aware of them for a long time, and have also warned the Indian government that the total cost incurred for the treatment of tobacco-related diseases exceeds the revenue acquired from the manufacture and sale of tobacco, by as much as Rs. 685 crores. This is a conservative estimate, and does not take into account the cost of establishing facilities for treatment. Besides these huge economic losses, tobacco addiction also causes human suffering, which cannot be translated into monetary terms. The Ministry of Health has accepted these findings and made a number of recommendations for effective tobacco control in India, similar to the Composite Tobacco Control Programme, enunciated by the World Health Organization. One of the significant provisions is that all tobacco products put up for sale, including bidis and chewing tobacco, should carry the health warning in two languages, English and Hindi or the regional language, and should depict the universally known danger sign, skull and crossbones, for non-literates.

The launching of the National Cancer Control Programme (NCCP) by the Ministry of Health and Family Welfare in 1985 gave an added impetus to tobacco control programmes in India. It led to the National Cancer Registry Project, and the establishment of Population-based and Hospital Cancer Registries. From the data obtained from these Registries, it was computed that about 48 per cent of cancers in men, and 20 per cent in women are due to tobacco habits. On an average, a third of all cancers in India are tobacco-related and entirely avoidable.

Two conferences, both held in Mumbai helped to focus attention on tobacco habits and tobacco-related diseases in India. The first one was a workshop 'Tobacco or Health', sponsored by the International Union Against Cancer (UICC) in April, 1987. The workshop brought together scientists, medical experts, policy makers, people working for voluntary organisations, and the media. They evaluated the available scientific evidence on possible hazards associated with various tobacco habits, and suggested suitable strategies for controlling them. One of the papers presented in this workshop revealed that Kerala has the highest number of tobacco addicts in India. About a lakh of foreign cigarettes flow into the state daily. It has the maximum number of registered bidi-workers' cooperatives, in addition to a number of independent bidi makers. Kerela is also one of the largest consumers of chewing tobacco. As expected, lung cancer is the most common cancer among men in Kerala. The worst feature is that lung cancer occurs in Kerala ten to fifteen years earlier than in developed countries. A reduction of age is seen in the incidence of coronary heart disease also.

Another conference, an international symposium on 'Control of Tobacco-related Cancers and Other Diseases', was held in January 1990 aspects of tobacco use were discussed.*

Many cancer hospitals and social workers are keenly interested in tobacco control programmes, and in increasing public awareness about the dangers of smoking. The Cancer Institute, Chennai, observes a '*no tobacco day*' every year. The Sundaram Medical Foundation in Chennai has adopted the '*can stop*' programme, aimed at ending smoking. The Indian Society on Tobacco and Health, whose members are medical and social workers, has been fighting tobacco addiction.

In Thiruvananthapuram, Kerala, the Regional Cancer Centre launched a massive programme using the help of college and high school

* The Proceedings of both these meetings have been published as *Tobacco and Health: The Indian Scene,* Eds. L.D. Sanghvi and P. Notani, UICC, , Tata Memorial Centre, Mumbai 1989; *Control of Tobacco-related Cancers and Other Diseases,* Eds. P.C. Gupta, J.E. Hamner III and P.R. Murti, Oxford University Press, Mumbai, 1992. Both of them together constitute a valuable source of information on tobacco habits in India, their health effects, and the dilemma faced by the government of India in implementing tobacco control measures.

students, health workers, voluntary agencies, social organisations, and the media, to combat the widespread tobacco addicion in Kerala. Under the National Service Scheme (N.S.S.), it has trained students from various colleges to carry out anti-smoking campaigns. High school students were educated on the evils of using tobacco. The students were rewarded for selling booklets on the harmful effects of tobacco. Health workers were trained to detect oral cancer and oral pre-cancers, and to create awareness among villagers about the harmful effects of chewing and smoking tobacco. This has enhanced primary prevention, and ensured early detection of oral cancers. Voluntary agencies and social organisations participated in all these anti-tobacco campaigns, carried out through lectures, slides and documentary films.

The Rajasthan Cancer Society has been vigorously campaigning against smoking in Jaipur and Jodhpur, through public lectures, distributing leaflets in the local language, slogans and slide shows. The Goa Cancer Society has been conducting health education camps for teachers and students in Sindhudurg and Ratnagiri, and has found that educating children often results in parents giving up smoking.

Some major national dailies have been regularly publishing articles on tobacco control and passive smoking. However, some of them also publish attractive colourful advertisements on cigarettes at the same time.

Recently, a lawsuit has been filed against cigarette companies, demanding that they compensate for the damages caused by smoking. It may not succeed, but it will succeed in focusing public attention on the harmful effects of smoking.

Recently, the Kerala High Court allowed two public interest writ petitions, and gave a judgment, banning smoking in 'public places in the state, like educational institutions, hospitals, commercial establishments, factories, cinema houses, walkways, bus stops and even railways stations'. Smoking in these areas will now be punishable under section 188 of the Indian Penal Code (IPC). A Division Bench of the High Court has said that, 'Public smoking is illegal, unconstitutional and is a violation of article 21 in the Constitution.' The judiciary has directed district collectors in the state to promulgate an order under Section 133(a) of the Criminal Procedure Code, prohibiting public smoking within a month from the date of the high court ruling. The office authorities have been asked to take appropriate steps to book the offenders. According to a Press Trust of India Report, the Hosdurg Magistrate Court in the Kasargod district, Kerala, has fined five people Rs. 500 each for smoking in public places. Two people who were unable to pay the fine, were imprisoned for fifteen days.

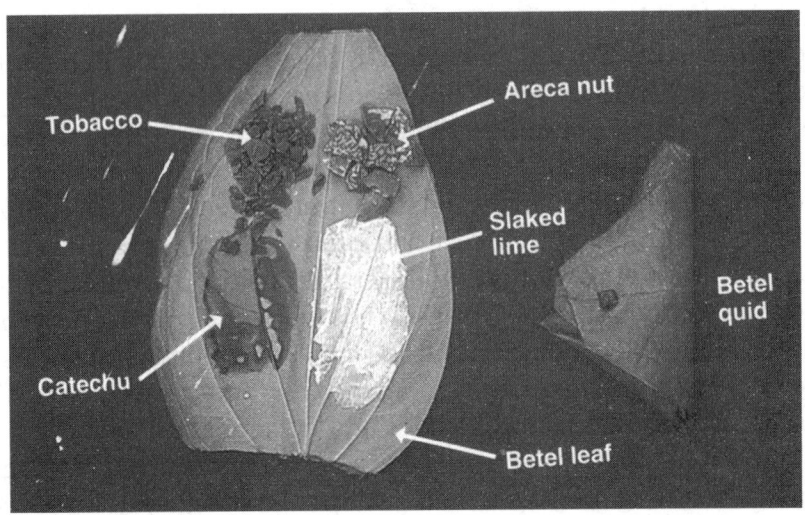

A betel quid preparation (Courtesy: Fali S Mehta, Head, Basic Dental Research Unit, Tata Institute of Fundamental Research, Mumbai)

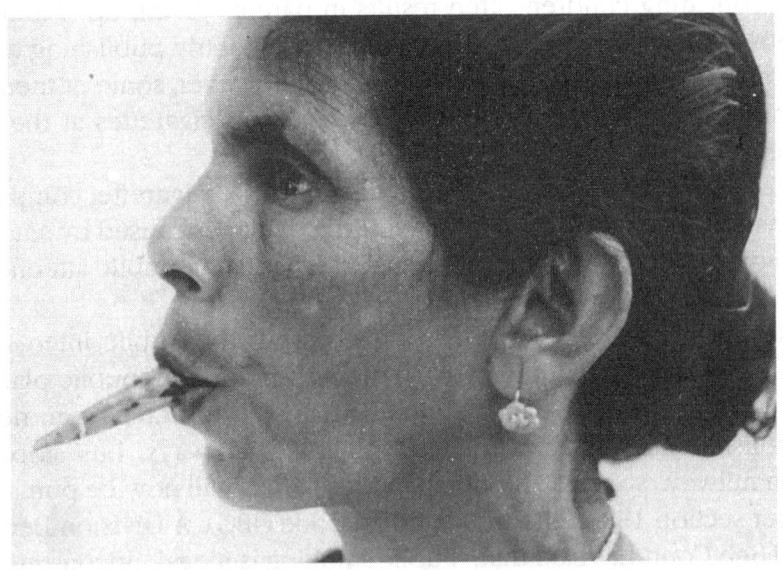

Reverse chutta smoking: a woman from Goa
(Courtesy: Fali S Mehta, Head, Basic Dental Research Unit,
Tata Institute of Fundamental Research, Mumbai)

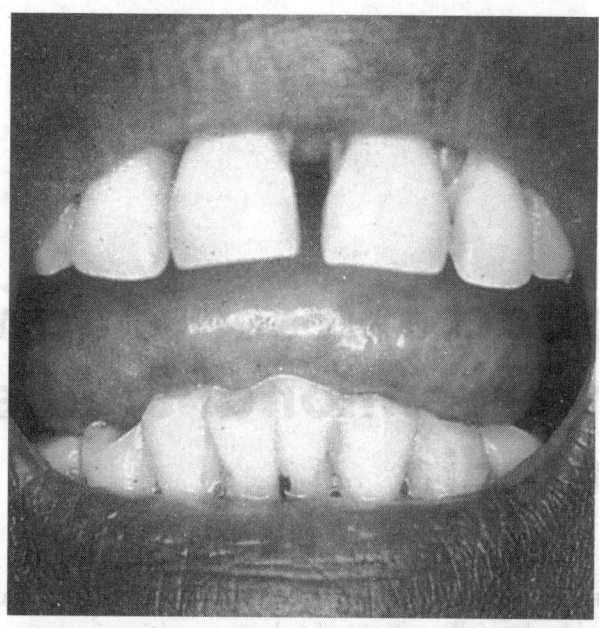

Submucous fibrosis. Note the shrunken tongue and difficulty in opening the mouth. (Courtesy: Fali S Mehta, Head, Basic Dental Research Unit, Tata Institute of Fundamental Research, Mumbai)

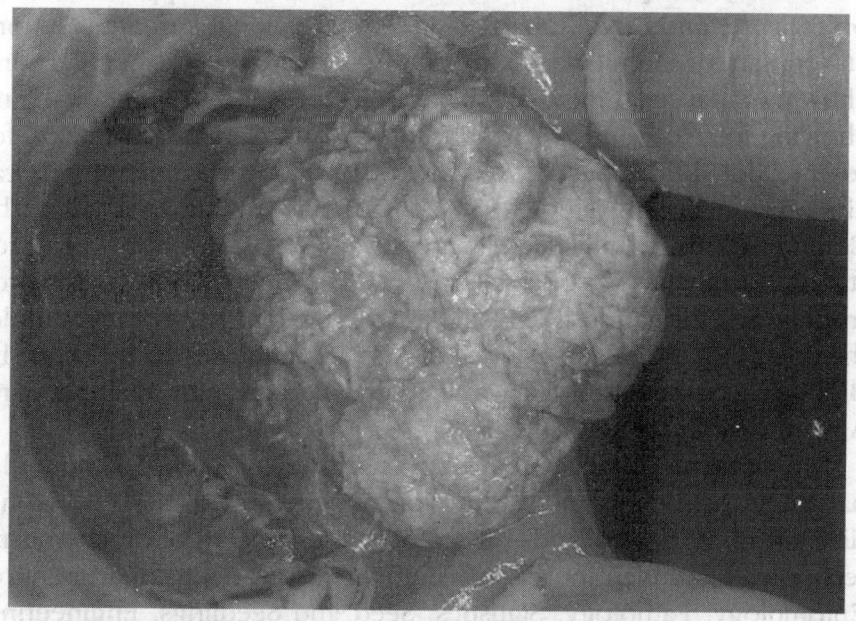

Cheek cancer in a betel quid chewer who also smoked (Courtesy: Fali S Mehta, Head, Basic Dental Research Unit, Tata Institute of Fundamental Research, Mumbai)

20 Tobacco Research and Interventional Studies in India

The Government of India set up the Indian Central Tobacco Committee in 1945, to develop all aspects of tobacco cultivation, processing, and marketing. The committee, in turn, established the Central Tobacco Research Institute at Rajahmundry, Andhra Pradesh, in 1947, to conduct fundamental research on all varieties of tobacco, and applied research on cigarette and Lanka tobaccos. It set up Regional Research Stations at Vedasandur (Tamil Nadu) in 1948 for research work on cigars and chewing tobacco; at Pusa (Bihar) in 1950, for research on hookah and chewing tobacco; and at Anand (Gujarat) and Nipani (Karnataka) for research on bidi tobacco. A cigarette tobacco research station was already functioning since 1936, at Guntur (Andhra Pradesh). The Committee also established a wrapper and hookah tobacco research station at Dinhatta (West Bengal) in 1952. The Central Tobacco Research Institute and the various Regional Research Stations were brought under the control of the Indian Council of Agricultural Research in 1965. The Bidi Tobacco Research Station at Anand became part of the Gujarat Agricultural University.

The **Central Tobacco Research Institute** (CTRI) in Rajahmundry has three main departments: division of genetics and plant breeding, division of agronomy and soil science, and division of biochemistry, technology and plant nutrition. There are also various departments of Entomology, Pathology, Statistics, Seed and Seedlings, Engineering; Farm Management. Keeping in mind the directive Scientific Coordination with which it was set up, the CTRI has involved itself with a variety of research projects, aiming to improve the quality, production and productivity of tobacco. It also studies factors that influence the quality of tobacco leaves produced, like colour of leaves (light or dark), texture (thin or heavy-bodied), elasticity, their nitrogen and nicotine contents, and their aroma and taste. The CTRI has acclimatised several exogenous varieties of tobacco to grow in India. Employing mutation, hybridisation and recombination techniques, it has also evolved new strains of tobacco like 'Kanakaprabha' and 'CTRI Special', which are of a better quality, have greater yield, are more pest-resistant, and so on.

Recently, with world opinion hardening against tobacco and tobacco addiction, the CTRI has embarked upon three new projects, which aim, to help tobacco control programmes. They are:

Product modification

This is an attempt to reduce the yield of tar and nicotine from cigarettes and bidis. It was found that adding potassium citrate to cigarette shreds, bring the potash level up to about 3.5 per cent, reduce the total particulate matter by 35 per cent, and bring down the mutagenicity of cigarette smoke by 80 per cent.

Scientists of the Gujarat Agricultural University at Anand have also carried out investigations to reduce the tar and nicotine yields of bidis. They have observed that 1. bidis made from all available varieties of tobaccos in India yield nearly the same levels of tar and nicotine, and 2. variations in growth conditions like transplanting dates, fertiliser nitrogen levels, source of nitrogen, irrigation, plant density, topping level and harvest date, do not produce tobacco with lower yields of nicotine and tar.

After testing three filters for bidis (cotton, cotton scented with amber and cigarette filters) they recommend the use of cotton scented with amber filters for bidis. It is effective in reducing the levels of toxic chemicals in the smoke, and is readily acceptable to consumers. When tobacco is grown in a carbon dioxide enriched atmosphere, the yield of leaves increased by 7 per cent. The leaves also contain less protein, nitrate, alkaloids and other chemicals which give rise to toxic substances like N-nitrosamines. Scientists at the Bidi Research Station at Anand are trying various strategies to grow tobacco under carbon dioxide enriched conditions.

Other uses of tobacco

Tobacco is a rich source of several phytochemicals like nicotine, solanesol organic acids (malic, citric and oxalic), and pentosans. About 10 per cent of the tobacco goes waste, when used in the manufacture of tobacco products like cigarettes and bidis. This serves as the material for manufacturing nicotine, solanesol, organic acids, and pentosans.

There are a few companies in Gujarat which make these chemicals from the bidi tobacco wastes.

Nicotine is widely used in the form of nicotine sulphate, as a pesticide. It also serves as the raw material for the manufacture of the pharmaceuticals, nicotinic acid and nicotinamide (found in the vitamin B complex), and nikhethamide. Solanesol is used as an intermediate for manufacturing a cardiac drug, and making vitamin K analogues. Malic and citric acids are used in both food and drug industries. Pentosans are used for production of the industrial solvent, furfural.

Roughly 40–42 per cent of tobacco seed comprises of oil. This is used as a semi-drying oil in the paint industry. When refined, it may also be used as edible oil. Proteins in the tobacco leaf can be useful as a food. Immature tobacco which is ninety days old, should be used to ensure the maximum extraction of all these chemicals.

Nicotine sulphate is a stomach, contact, and fumigant poison. It is widely used as an insecticide in orchards in Japan. Both nicotine sulphate and solanesol are exported to Japan, the U.K, the U.S.A., Canada, Switzerland and Germany. There is thus a good export market for both these chemicals. The possibility of utilising nicotine sulphate as a pesticide in India itself should be explored. As a natural product, it may have advantages over synthetic pesticides that we use at present.

Substitute crops for tobacco

The feasibility of growing other crops remuneratively instead of tobacco, has been explored. However there are many inherent difficulties in arriving at a possible solution. Tobacco is a drought-tolerant, rugged plant, and can grow in semi-arid areas. It is also resistant to many pests, and is a remunerative cash crop for farmers. Most other plants do not possess these qualities. Andhra Pradesh and Gujarat tried in vain to substitute tobacco with cotton and chillies. Cotton is not resistant to many pests, and gives low yields. Chickpeas, mustard, coriander and safflower, can be successfully grown instead of FCV tobacco on the black soils of Andhra Pradesh but their market prices are subject to great fluctuation. Hence, farmers prefer to grow only tobacco, which gives a more steady income.

In Gujarat, castor can be grown more remuneratively, but the demand for castor oil has not been assessed so far. In West Bengal, crops like potato, cauliflower and mustard are more remunerative than the cigar filler and chewing tobacco cultivated there. However, these crops sometimes fetch very low prices due to overproduction. In Tamil Nadu chillies, safflower, groundnut or cotton can easily substitute the chewing tobacco grown rotationally between bajra, ragi, and sorghum. Farmers, however, still prefer to grow tobacco because of the erratic monsoon pattern which will bring varying yields with he o her crops. Bihar is the only place, where chewing toba. co is stea dv giving place to sugarcane, maize, potatoes, groundnut, an i mu .a'd.

The investigations carried out at variou s tob;.cco research stations thus reveal the possibilities and problem, connected with:

- ❑ Product modification, aimed at re ducin g tar and nicotine yields of cigarettes and bidis;
- ❑ Alternate uses of tobacco, with the v irious chemicals that can be manufactured from it; and
- ❑ Substituting other crops for t)bacc) in the tobacco cultivated areas of India.

EPIDEMIOLOGICAL INVESTIGATIONS AND LABORATORY ANALYSIS

Epidemilogical studies on cancer in India are now nearly a century old. As early as 1902, Niblock observed an appreciable number of oral cancer patients in the Government General Hospital at Chennai. He correctly ascribed this to the prevailing betel quid and tobacco chewing habits among the people. A more detailed case-control study was carried out by O.r in 1933 among the people of Travancore (now known as Kerala), which confirmed Niblock's observation, and clearly established betel quid along with tobacco addiction as the cause for oral cancer.

Wahi and co-workers have carried out extensive studies on tobacco habits in the Mainpuri district of Uttar Pradesh in 1965–66. Tobacco is mixed with slaked lime, finely-cut areca nut, camphor, and cloves. About 7 per cent of the villagers are addicted to this preparation. Prolonged chewing is found to lead initially to leukoplakia and oral submucous fibrosis and later on to oral and oropharyngeal cancers. Smoking and chewing tobacco, combined with alcohol consumption is found to increase the risk for these cancers synergistically.

In 1959, Shanta and Krishnamurthi studied the etiological factors causing oral cancer (squamous cell cancer). A sharp increase in all tobacco-related cancers in Chennai during the period 1987–91 compared to 1982–86, has been reported by Gajalakshmi, Ravichandran and Shanta in 1996. The per capita consumption of tobacco has also increased during this period. A survey of 7,737 households in Chennai, conducted during 1997–98, revealed that among men, the proportion of smoking, chewing and drinking alcohol were 31.1 per cent, 7 per cent and 10 per cent respectively; eight per cent of women chewed tobacco, but hardly any of them smoked or drank; about 88 per cent were aware of the harmful effects of smoking and chewing tobacco.

A case-control study carried out by Sanghvi, Rao and Khanolkar in 1955 at the Tata Memorial Centre, Mumbai, revealed that smoking bidis leads to cancers of the oral cavity, pharynx, larynx, and esophagus, and contribute largely to cancers at the oropharynx; and chewing tobacco, besides leading to oral cancer, contributes to cancers of the larynx, pharynx, and esophagus. These results were later independently confirmed by Jussawalla and Deshpande.

Bidi smoke was chemically analysed only in 1974 by Hoffmann, Sanghvi, and Wynder in the U.S.A. laboratory and was found to contain larger amounts of toxic chemicals like tar, nicotine, carbon monoxide, and hydrogen cyanide than cigarette smoke. This suggests that smoking bidis is far more dangerous than smoking cigarettes. An analysis of smoke from various brands of bidis has been carried out since then in India, by Pakhale and co-workers at the Cancer Research Institute, Mumbai. Most of the tobacco used in India contain a higher percentage of nicotine than tobacco used in the West. Also, the tobacco used for making bidis is considerably richer in nicotine than the tobacco blend used in making cigarettes. This explains the higher yield of nicotine from bidis, though they contain only a fraction of the tobacco used in cigarettes. The carcinogenicity of bidi smoke was confirmed by Bhide, who observed that seven out of fifteen BALB/c mice treated with bidi smoke, condensate developed tumours (one gastric carcinoma, one esophageal cancer, four liver haemangiomas, and one papilloma of the stomach).

Recent investigations by Bhisey and co-workers suggest that the vast number of women rolling bidis, constantly inhale tobacco dust and hence have a high risk of tobacco-related diseases. The urine of bidi rollers was found to contain cotinine as well as thioethers, revealing the cutaneous and lung absorption of nicotine and other toxic components of tobacco.

Investigation by Nagabhusan and co-workers reveal that betel leaves by themselves are anti-mutagenic and anti-carcinogenic, and will tend to counteract the carcinogenicity of tobacco. Catechu has also been found to be anti-mutagenic.

Interventional studies

Cross-sectional studies carried out by Mehta and co-workers among 4,000 Bombay policemen in 1960–61 revealed that there is an appreciable incidence of leukoplakia and oral cancer among paan chewers and bidi smokers. A survey carried out in 1965–66 by Pindborg and co-workers among 35,000 outpatients in dental clinics in Bangalore, Lucknow, Bombay and Trivandrum confirmed the high prevalence of leukoplakia in India.

These studies led to a large scale, marathon project on oral cancer and pre-cancers, carried out by the Basic Dental Research Unit of the Tata Institute of Fundamental Research, Mumbai. The project, supported entirely by funds from the National Institutes of Health, U.S.A. under the P.L. 480 Indo-American Research Agreement, lasted for twenty-seven years, and began in 1966. Dr Fali S Mehta of the Basic Dental Research Unit served as the Principal Investigator; the late Dr. Jens J. Pindborg of the Department of Oral Pathology, Royal Dental College, Copenhagen, Denmark, as the co-principal investigator; and Dr. James E. Hamer III, from the University of Tennessee, as the N.I.H. project officer. Some of the other investigators involved in this project were Drs. P.R. Murti, R.B. Bhonsle, P.N. Senor and D.K. Daftary (all Dentists); Dr Prakash C. Gupta (Statistics), and Dr. Mira B. Aghi.

A unique feature of the project, was that it was a population-based, house to house survey in the rural areas, and involved as many as 2,00,000 subjects. In terms of persons involved, money spent, and the duration, it was one of the largest projects ever carried out in India so far. Though expensive, and time-consuming, the project yielded rich dividends and for the first time provided, an integrated picture of the various tobacco habits in India. It has also given a lot of information on the pathogenesis of the pre-cancers, leukoplakia and oral submucous fibrosis and palatal lesions, and the subsequent onset of oral and palatal cancers, mainly from the pre-cancers. Above all, it has demonstrated the feasibility of intervention through health education, resulting in a 'significant and substantial' decrease in oral pre-cancers and cancer.

In the first phase of the project, lasting from 1966–69, a survey of the prevalence of various tobacco habits among villagers in seven select areas of India was carried out. The areas selected were Ernakulam in Kerala, Goa, Pune, Bhavnagar in Gujarat, Srikakulam in Andhra Pradesh, Singhbhum and Darbhanga in Bihar. The survey revealed that bidi smoking was most common among men in all these places, except Srikakulam, where chutta and reverse chutta smoking were practised. Cigarette smoking was high only in Kerala, among 6 per cent of the population. In Bhavnagar, Srikakulam, and Goa, most men smoked. Chewing was more common in Pune and Uttar Pradesh while in Ernakulam, Singhbhum, Darbhanga and Mainpuri, both smoking and chewing were widely practised. Women preferred chewing tobacco to smoking in all the places except Srikaklam, where almost all of them practised reverse chutta smoking and in Duarbhanga, where hookah smoking was more common. This study revealed that tobacco use in one form or other is quite common in rural India, ranging from

61 per cent (Pune) to 88 per cent (Andhra Pradesh) among men; and 15 per cent (Goa) to 67 per cent (Srikakulam) among women.

A survey of 50,915 villagers in four states revealed twenty-six cases of oral cancer. The prevalence of leukoplakia ranged from 0.2–4.9 per cent and mainly affected men. Leukoplakia was found to strike at a younger age than oral cancer. Its starts appearing among people of the 15–24 age group, and to a larger extent in the 25–34 age group. The exact location of the leukoplakia depended very much on the kind of chewing and smoking practised. Hookli smoking led to leukoplakia on the labial mucosa, and reverse chutta smoking on the palate. Epithelial atypia was seen in 8.4 per cent of homogeneous leukoplakia, but in 59.1 per cent of speckled leukoplakias. Submucous fibrosis occured exclusively among betel quid and areca nut chewers, areca nut being the etiological factor. It strikes mainly in the oral cavity and occasionally, in the pharynx and oropharynx.

A ten-year follow up study of this population revealed that:

❐ Preleukoplakia and leukoplakia occurred only among those who smoked or chewed tobacco

❐ Oral cancer occurred almost always from the pre-cancers, leukoplakia, or submucous fibrosis; and

❐ While leukoplakia may regress, after a person stopped consuming tobacco, submucous fibrosis, once formed, does not regress at all. It is definitely a pre-cancerous state.

In a seventeen-year follow up of sixty-six cases of oral submucous fibrosis, oral cancer developed in 0.4 per cent of cases at the end of ten years; in 4.5 per cent at the end of fifteen years, and in 7.6 per cent at the end of seventeen years. Only if one stops chewing tobacco, can one prevent its further transformation into oral cancer. Other oral lesions like leukedema, leukokeratosis, nicotina palati, palatal erythema, central papillary atrophy of the tongue, paan chewer's lesion or oral lichen planus-like lesion do not become malignant. Reverse chutta smoking led to a variety of palatal changes like keratosis, excrescences, patches, red areas, ulcerations and non-pigmented areas. Red areas are the most dangerous, with 52 per cent of them exhibiting epithelial dysplasia.

Over a ten-year follow up period, ten cases of palatal cancers arose, all from pre-existing red areas or patches. The majority of palatal lesions, about 75 per cent remained as they were, while a small percentage (14 per cent) underwent regression. The palatal lesions regressed further if a person stoped smoking. Thus, the ten-year follow up study revealed that oral cancer and oral pre-cancers occur only among tobacco addicts, showing that the abolition of smoking and chewing tobacco should reduce incidence of oral cancer.

The third phase of the project was the actual 'intervention' which attempted to investigate firstly, whether health education could motivate tobacco users into giving up tobacco, and secondly, determining the impact on the oral pre-cancers. A ten-year prospective study (1977–86) was conducted in three areas – Ernakulam, Srikakulam and Bhavnagar. Each place built an 'intervention cohort' constituting about 12,000 people, who were periodically trained on how to quit tobacco. A control cohort of about 10,000 tobacco users was formed from the previous ten-year study. These people did not receive any or only minimal levels of health education. It was seen that most tobacco users began using tabacco, believing it to have medicinal value, such as, a curative for toothache, bad breath and gastric disturbances. Some were vaguely aware that tobacco was harmful but very few knew all about its deleterious effects. In the Bhavnagar district, only men were targeted, as very few women smoked or chewed tobacco.

The intervention team consisted of dentists, trained social workers, interviewing clerks, and locals. At the beginning of this stage, all the subjects were examined by dentists. People in the intervention cohort were then offered medical advice, and educated on the need for, and method used, to stop tobacco consumption. They were also informed of the withdrawal symptoms through individual or group interviews. Personal communication helped clarify doubts and clear individual problems relating to tobacco use. Confidence and trust were also built up through these sessions. At each one-year follow up, the subjects were asked about their tobacco habits, to see if there was any reduction. They were than examined by the dentists for any possible pre-cancerous changes. This was followed with encouragement to maintain or intensify the motivation to quit. Each annual follow up thus assessed the efficacy of the intervention phase. In addition to personal advice, a variety of other strategies were employed to make the intervention effective. Films were found to be effective in bringing about behavioural changes, particularly as the intervention population included non-literates and semi-literates. Being a mass media, films had the advantage of communicating to a large audience at one time. Specially designed posters, some with written messages, and others with pictures, were used to remind the target population of the need to quit tobacco consumption. Slides prepared from these posters, were shown in the nearby theatres. Folk dramas which were found to be very popular in the Srikakulam area, were effective in conveying the message against tobacco use. Radio programmes in the form of talks, interviews, dramas, and documentaries, and articles in local newspapers, were also used to educate the public. Finally, cessation camps were held to help those who had made previous attempts to quit tobacco consumption but were unable to do so. Thus, all conceivable methods were employed to bring about behavioural changes in tobacco users.

The intervention trials were found to be very effective in both Ernakulam and Srikakulam. In Ernakulam, at the end of the intervention, about 14 per cent of tobacco users have completely stopped usage, and many others have significantly reduced their tobacco consumption. This has brought about a decrease in the leukoplakia rate in Ernakulam, and palatal changes in Srikakulam, which, in turn, would signify a decrease in the rampancy of cancers. However, the intervention trials in Bhavnagar had no significant effect on the tobacco habits of that population.

PROTECTIVE AGENTS AGAINST SMOKING AND CHEWING TOBACCO

Oral cancer is a major health problem in Kerala. An attempt has been made by the Regional Cancer Centre, Thiruvananthapuram, to elucidate the risk factors for cancers at specific sites within the oral cavity. It was observed that chewing betel quid containing tobacco increases the risk of cancers in the buccal mucosa and the gingivum. This is explained by the fact that the people in this part of India customarily keep the bolus of betal quid in between the buccal cavity and gingivum.

Smoking is found to be the major cause of cancer in the anterior two-thirds of the tongue.

As there is a high prevalence of oral leukoplakia in Kerala because of the high betel quid consumption rate, investigations have been carried out to see whether chemoprevention of leukoplakia is possible. Chemoprevention is a form of primary prevention, by taking in dietary or pharmacological inhibitors of carcinogenesis. Investigations were conducted on fishermen who had oral leukoplakias because of chewing betel quid. About 65 per cent of these participants also drank, while 30 per cent were bidi smokers. Treatment with oral vitamin A as retinyl acetate at a level of 300,000 I.U. per week for a year, causes complete regression of leukoplakias in 52 per cent of the cases. Beta carotene at 360 mg per week for a year effected a complete regression in a third of the cases, while only 10 per cent of regression was observed in placebos. The fishermen continued smoking, chewing and drinking throughout the treatment period. Homogeneous leukoplakias and smaller lesions responded more readily than non-homogeneous and larger lesions. No toxicity was observed but a relapse occurred when the supplementation with vitamin A or beta carotene was stopped. Vitamin A was found to be more effective than beta carotene. These investigations reveal that chemoprevention of the incidence of oral leukoplakias can be achieved through administration of vitamin A or beta carotene, even when the tobacco habits are being continued. The success rate however, is not very high.

Other contributions

Both basic and clinical research on various aspects of smoking and chewing tobacco are continuing in several laboratories in India. Statistics on the morbidity and mortality due to smoking and chewing tobacco, have been compiled earlier by Gupta of the Tata Institute of Fundamental Research, Mumbai, and Jayant and Notani of the Tata Memorial Centre. Information on cancer incidence, morbidity and mortality are available from the reports of the National Cancer Registry Project. The use of hand-held computers (electronic diaries) for numbering tobacco addicts among the general population in big cities like Mumbai, has recently been reported by Gupta of the Tata Institute of Fundamental Research.

21 Considerations, Suggestions and Future Prospects

There are more diverse tobacco consumption habits in India than in any other country in the world. Bidis and cigarettes are the most common forms of smoking in India, while cigars, cheroots, chuttas, and reverse chuttas, hookahs, hooklis, and chillums are less common. Besides the cancers caused by cigarettes, smoking bidi leads to a higher incidence of cancers in the pharynx, larynx, and the base of the tongue; reverse chutta smoking, causes cancer in the hard palate. Thus, the resulting cancers are equally varied.

The chewing habits are equally diverse in India. Plain tobacco with slaked lime, other tobacco preparations (khaini, zarda, kiwam, Mainpuri), a variety of areca nut preparations (raw areca nut slices, fermented areca nut (bura tammool); scented areca nut (supari), mawa, paan masala, paan masala gutka), and betel quid in various combinations are chewed. In addition, a variety of tobacco preparations (mishri, bajjar, gudhaku, and creamy snuff toothpaste) are used as dentifrices. All these result in very high rates of oral cancer, and cause pre-cancers, leukoplakia and oral submucous fibrosis.

Chewing also causes cancers of the pharynx, larynx, and esophagus. In the West, cancers of the mouth, larynx and pharynx together constitute 5–10 per cent of the total cancers. However, they are all serious health problems in India, accounting for 30–40 per cent of all cancers among men in some places.

BIDI

The bidi is now the most common form of smoking and of tobacco use in the country. It is a tobacco product unique to India, and yields greater amounts of tar and nicotine than cigarette. Epidemiological investigations show that it also causes cancers of the pharynx, larynx, and of the posterior third of the tongue. It is undoubtedly responsible, at least in part, for the relatively far higher incidence of these cancers in India.

However, any attempt to reduce bidi consumption must be carefully planned, since the manufacture and marketing of bidis provides employment to over three million people. However the government can make a small beginning by insisting on 'health warnings' on all packets of bidis and chewing tobaccos. It can also insist on bidis being provided with cotton filters, scented with amber so that the tar and nicotine yields of bidis are reduced. This may make the bidi slightly more expensive, but the resulting health benefits will more than compensate for it.

CIGARETTE

Cigarette smoking is likely to increase rapidly in India in the future. There is only a limited ban on cigarette advertising so that cigarette manufacturing companies can use aggressive marketing tactics to promote their products. Cigarettes are more common among affluent students especially male students who are low achievers. Very few girls smoke at present.

While cigarettes in all the developed countries, yield low amounts of tar and nicotine, their yield from Indian cigarettes is still very high (19–20 mg of tar, and aboout 2 mg of nicotine per cigarette).

Even, the so-called filter cigarettes in India have high tar and nicotine yield. Both the Indian government, and the Consumer Council of India should act against this immediately. In many Western countries, cigarette companies have to print the tar and nicotine yields on cigarette packets. The ministry of health, of the Indian government should also consider implementing this.

The large-scale entry of multinational cigarette companies into India will result in a continuous drain on foreign exchange, besides ruining the health of the nation. The only factor which prevents a greater use of cigarettes in India is an availability of the bidi as a cheap substitute. As India 'progresses', the cigarette may replace the bidi.

HOOKAH

Hookah smoking which began during the mughal period, is still practised in the Middle East. India exports substantial amounts of hookah paste to countries in this region.

Nicotine

The long-term harmful effects of cigarette smoking have been known for over forty years now. However, people in all countries still continue to smoke. This is because of the profound psychological effects exerted by nicotine, which is reported to improve learning and memory in the individuals.

The question arises whether nicotine alone can be used safely to produce the desired psychological effect. At the moment, it is used as nicotine patches, nicotine chewing gum, or spray, primarily to control withdrawal effects.

Nicotine's known adverse effects are on the cardiovascular system. If we could find a cardioprotective agent which will protect the vascular system, without interfering with the psychological and other desirable effects of nicotine, then it could be used for a number of purposes, including treatment of Parkinson's and allied diseases. It will also enable the development of a really 'safe cigarette', without any cardiotoxicity.

Areca nut

The areca nut is extremely popular in India and is chewed in a variety of ways. Unfortunately, some of the preparations are harmful, causing diseases such as oral submucous fibrosis. This is a serious ailment, characterised by a strong rigidity of the oral mucosa (loss of elasticity). In extreme cases, the person may not be able to open her mouth at all. This condition does not regress, and in some cases can develop into oral cancer. There is no known cure for oral submucous fibrosis. A survey revealed that about 10.9 per cent of mawa chewers were suffering from oral submucous fibrosis. Many of them were young, well below thirty-five years; they had begun chewing mawa at an early age. The mechanism of how the areca nut induces submucous fibrosis should be studied and also, whether it could be prevented by simultaneously chewing a protective agent.

Paan masala and gutka are well-advertised popular areca nut preparations chewed in northern India. Gutka also contains tobacco. Many eipidemiologists and dentists fear that these will lead to high rates of oral submucous fibrosis and oral cancer in the future.

The areca nut is potentially carcinogenic. It contains alkaloids, which can undergo nitrosation changes inside the body to give rise carcinogenic N-nitrosamines. An epidemiological report from Natal in South Africa, states that habitual chewing of areca nut **alone** by Indian women there, has led to oral cancer.

'Bura tammool' which is often fungus-infected may or may not have contributed to the very high incidences of pharyngeal and esophageal cancers prevalent there.

While tobacco has been extensively studied, there is still scope for research work on the biological effects of areca nut, and of various preparations containing areca nut. There are also innumerable imitations sold as areca nut in small packets in wayside shops in Chennai, and consumed by the public, without knowing its contents. Both the Consumer Council of India and the state government should thoroughly investigate what these packets contain, and their biological effects.

BETEL QUID (PAAN)

Epidemiological studies suggest that betel quid without tobacco does not pose a significant risk of cancer. Among the various components of paan, the individual ones betel leaves protect against carcinogenesis areca nut could induce cancer, and chunam (slaked lime), an irritant could act as a promoter. Hence, habitual chewers would do well to increase the number of betel leaves, minimise the quantities of areca nut and slaked lime, and strictly avoid tobacco. The frequency of chewing should also be restricted.

Nationwide survey
Unfortunately, we do not have a nationwide aurvey of tobacco, betel quid and areca nut habits in India. A population-based nationwide survey will be very expensive; but will provide a wealth of baseline information, on which other studies can be based. Though a nationwide survey does not exist, considerable information is available from other sources, which include:
1. The project on oral cancer and pre-cancers, carried out for twenty-seven years by the Basic Dental Research Unit of the Tata Institute of Fundamental Research, Mumbai, in six districts in India (Ernakulam; Pune; Srikakulam; Bhavnagar; Singhbhum; and Darbhanga) from 1966 to 1993;
2. The population based Cancer Registries at Chennai, Bangalore, Mumbai, Ahmedabad, Delhi, Bhopal, and Barshi;
3. The Hospital Cancer Registries at Thiruvanathapuram and Dibrugarh; and
4. Various research papers published from cancer and other centres at different times.

All the information thus gathered, makes it possible to build up an integrated picture of smoking and chewing habits in India.

The role of the government of India
The Government of India should declare unequivocally that complete tobacco control within India is its ultimate goal. It must work out a

long-term plan to erase tobacco addiction in stages. It should also take into full consideration its own finances, including its astronomical foreign debt, and the various economic and social issues involved. A practical policy at this juncture would be a mixture of both tobacco promotion and tobacco control.

India earns a substantial amount of foreign exchange by exporting FCV and other varieties of tobacco, and tobacco products like hookah paste, zarda, as well as small amounts of cigarettes and bidis. In view of its foreign debt it is imperative that India increase its exports. It should be remembered that even the U.K. and U.S.A., which are strictly and successfully implementing tobacco control programmes at home, have not cut down on their cigarette manufacture nor have they stopped dumping them in third world countries. India would do well to export high quality products which are less harmful.

The Tobacco Board should also increase the manufacture and export of other tobacco products like the pesticides, nicotine sulphate, vitamins, nicotinic acid, and nicotinamide, the pharmaceutical intermediate solanesol, and tobacco seed oil. At present, only one or two factories in Gujarat are manufacturing these products. The Central Tobacco Research Institute has suggested the possibility of using tobacco seed protein as an edible protein. This has to be tested first through animal experiments, for toxicity and nutritive value.

In order to bring about effective tobacco control, the Indian government should enforce, through appropriate legislation:
1. The maximum permissible values for tar and nicotine yields of cigarettes, (15 mg tar and 1 mg nicotine per cigarette as adopted by the European Union). Cigarettes yielding higher amounts should be taxed heavily. This will automatically make the cigarette companies conform to the permitted values. Selling filter cigarettes (that are more expensive but yield the same or higher amounts of tar and nicotine) rather than ordinary cigarettes is nothing short of cheating the customers and should be made a punishable offence.

Chewing tobacco and bidi packets should carry health warnings. Bidis should also be provided with effective filters.

There should be a strict ban on tobacco and cigarette advertising throughout the country.

The sale of cigarettes and bidis to minors should be banned.
None of these measures will affect the revenue to the Government of India.

It is estimated that about 30 per cent of cigarettes in any country are smuggled, causing the government to lose that amount of revenue. The Government of India should safeguard against smuggling.

Companies allege that the high taxes and consequent high prices of cigarettes, are reasons why smuggling occurs. It may thus be necessary to optimise the tax on cigarettes.

Dr. Nigel Gray, an advocate of the anti-smoking campaign in Australia, repeatedly warns that, 'Multinational cigarette companies should never be allowed to enter or establish themselves in any country. The huge profits made by them will cause a continuous foreign exchange drain'.

The state governments should provide more remunerative jobs for bidi workers as alternatives

It should also seriously consider reports of dentists, that a habitual consumption of paan masala and gutka leads to oral submucous fibrosis and other oral lesions.

There should be a radical change in the attitude of Indian society towards smoking, if any tobacco control programme is to succeed. Smoking is now an accepted practice in society.

Indians are only vaguely aware that smoking can injure one's health; very few know how smoking can actually harm a person. Hence, any tobacco control programme should begin by educating the public, about the debilitating effects of smoking. The medical profession and the media can do this best, doctors can be invited to talk to large gatherings, or on television, or radio. Anti-smoking messages in cinemas, could be one of the most powerful means of reaching the masses.

Popular English and regional language dailies should also be inducted in the campaign for non-smoking. *The Hindu*, a widely read popular English daily, is already pioneering a campaign against smoking in south India. It publishes regular articles on the adverse effects of active and passive smoking, on the punishments meted out to offenders who smoke in public places, and so on.

Quitting smoking

Smoking is a difficult habit to quit, once it becomes addictive. An intensive cessation therapy produced a quit rate of only 35 per cent, implying that the rest were unable to quit smoking.

Similar results were obtained at the end of the Interventional Trials by the Basic Dental Research Unit of the Tata Institute of Fundamental Research, in Ernakulam, Kerala. In spite of administering various intervention techniques like personal communication, documentary films, radio talks, folk plays, and cessation camps, for ten years, only 14 per cent of the addicts completely stopped using tobacco, though some reduced their frequency of tobacco use. These studies lasting for twenty-seven years have, undoubtedly, produced a wealth of information on the prevalence of various tobacco and areca nut habits in this district, and on the pathogenesis of leukoplakia, oral submucous fibrosis and oral cancer. But, as an intervention, it was not a great success. Once again, the same conclusion is reached: The tobacco habit, whether smoking or chewing, is difficult to quit. It is best not to start the habit.

A strong motivation is absolutely necessary for a person to stop consuming tobacco. The addict could also use various aids, like nicotine chewing gum, nicotine patches, and nicotine spray. The Central Tobacco Research Institute can develop methods for their manufacture in our own country. A press report published by the WHO claimed that it would make these products available at subsidised rates. Private 'smoking cessation clinics' have started coming up in our country. As they are likely to be very expensive, often beyond the means of the average smoker, it may be better, if such clinics are started in government hospitals. Smokers can also form self-help groups.

Protective agents

Forty years of attempting tobacco control has revealed that, firstly, tobacco habits will persist, and cannot be eliminated overnight, and secondly, they can be reduced only marginally, as revealed by intervention trials. These disappointing findings led to a third approach as to whether tobacco could be prevented from exerting its harmful health effects, by simultaneously administering a protective agent. This is known as chemoprevention, preventing tobacco's harmful effects, by counteracting it with a protective agent. Drs. Krishnan Nair, Sankara Narayanan, and others in the Regional Cancer Centre, Trivandrum, have investigated the effects of administering vitamin A or beta carotene to fishermen, who regularly chewed betel quid. As many as 65 per cent also drank alcohol, and 30 per cent smoked bidis. Vitamin A was found to prevent the incidence of oral leukoplakia in 52 per cent of the cases, and beta carotene, in 33 per cent. These investigations reveal that chemoprevention is at least partially effective.

We have conducted experiments on chemoprevention of cancer in laboratory animals. We have observed that the induction of gastric cancer in Swiss mice by the potent carcinogen, 3, 4 benzo(a)pyrene; and hepatomas in Wistar rats by 3'-methyl 4-dimethylam inoazobenzene, can be effectively prevented by the simultaneous feeding of cumin seeds (jeera). Poppy seeds (khuskhus), basil leaves (tulasi) and ponnakanni leaves have also been found to be effective, but to a lesser extent. Various other scientists have shown that turmeric is also anti-carcinogenic. As we are not likely to eliminate or reduce smoking or chewing in the near future, the possibility of preventing their adverse health effects by consuming these plant products holds great promise. Further work on these lines with dietary components as protective agents should be carried out. Investigators in the West have found that regular consumption of yellow-green fruits and vegetables reduces significantly the incidence of breast cancer and heart diseases.

Kerala's experience

Kerala has the highest rates of tobacco addiction in India, though it does not grow any tobacco. It is a major producer of areca nuts and supplies it in a variety of forms (kotapakku, kalipakku, seeval) to other states. The detailed surveys, investigations, and interventions carried out by the Basic Dental Research Unit of the T.I.F.R. in Ernakulam District for over twenty-seven years show that, Kerala, probably has the highest incidence of oral cancer in India, among both men and women. It is also the state, where the first case-control studies confirming betel quid tobacco chewing as the root cause of oral cancer, was carried out by Orr in 1933. The Regional Cancer Centre at Thiruvananthapuram is presently carrying out a wide range of research projects on oral cancer and leukoplakia and their control, with the help of international funding. Kerala has taken the initiative in banning smoking in public places.

The future

It is predicted that deaths due to tobacco consumption for the whole world will increase from the present level of three million to about ten million by the year 2025, out of which a death rate of seven million will be from the developing countries. China alone will account for two million deaths. At present, deaths caused by tobacco addiction in India, is estimated between 630,000 and one million. It is likely to be higher in the future, because of increasing cigarette consumption, and increased longevity. India may thus account for another two million deaths by 2025. Lung cancer, which is a good indicator of smoking behaviour addiction has been steadily increasing at all places in India, as reported by Cancer Registries. Some epidemiologists have predicted a lung cancer epidemic in India, if the present trend continues.

Many countries in Asia are now initiating precautionary measures against the long-term ill-effects of tobacco consumption. China, Malaysia, Hong Kong, Korea and Thailand have established national coordinating organisations on tobacco control. Singapore and Thailand have enacted very strict laws on smoking and tobacco control, and are enforcing them too. The Ministry of Health, Government of India, has recommended a wide range of measures for tobacco control in India; but only some of them have been put into practice. On the whole, India's approach to tobacco control has been half-hearted so far. Public opinion against tobacco use in India is yet to gather momentum.

Smoking will continue to decline steadily in the U.K. and U.S.A., during the coming years. There will be a progressive decrease in mortality due to tobacco-related diseases. But, it is very doubtful, if these countries will be able to completely eradicate smoking. There is a growing public opinion the world over, particularly among health lobbyists that, these countries should restrict the multinational cigarette companies to follow certain definite norms. The U.S. and U.K. tobacco companies and their subsidiaries should adhere to the same standards of product, marketing, promotion and sales in developing countries, as are required in their own countries. They should also stop pressurising governments in developing countries to prevent passing and implementation of anti-tobacco measures. It has been alleged that some U.S. senators and U.S. consulates help these tobacco companies in their export and cigarette promotional activities. In the long run, the U.S. and U.K. governments will earn the goodwill of the whole world, if they put an end to the dumping of cigarettes in third world countries.

The high prevalence of oral cancer in different regions of India has been reported by several investigators from time to time. In Singapore, the incidence of oral cancer among Indians is considerably greater than among Chinese or Malay residents there. Indians in Malaysia account for 52 per cent of the oral cancer admissions although they form only 10 per cent of the Malaysian population. Oral cancer and oral submucous fibrosis are common among the Indian community in Natal, South Africa. The reason for the high prevalence of oral cancer is the practice of chewing betel quid with tobacco.

It is well-known that chewing tobacco leads to various oral lesions, including oral cancer. The advent of paan masala, an areca nut preparation, has led to a vast increase in oral submucous fibrosis. The epidemiogical investigations among Indian women in Natal, South Africa have some common features. About 50 per cent of the women who chew the areca nut, do so without using tobacco or betel quid.

Oral submucous fibrosis occurred in 38 per cent of the people, especially in those who chewed areca nut without betel quid. Oral cancer among women occurred mainly in the buccal mucosa and tongue and 65 per cent of these cancers arose in women who did not use any tobacco. This South African investigation clearly demonstrates that chewing areca nut, alone can lead to oral submucous fibrosis and oral cancer. The messages from all these findings are clear. Chewing of tobacco should be avoided, as it undoubtedly leads to oral cancer. Habitual chewing of areca nut and areca nut preparations like paan masala carry a high risk of oral submucous fibrosis and oral cancer, and are therefore best avoided. Areca nut is an integral part of betel quid. Hence, betel quid should contain only a minimum amount of areca nut and no tobacco. It is safer to use such betel quid, for this does not carry any significant risk for oral cancer. As an educated community, we should restrict ourselves only to safe betel quids; our unenviable reputation of having the highest oral cancer rates, will then be a thing of the past.

Index